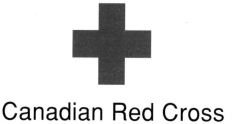

Canadian Red Cross

First Aid & CPR Manual

This manual belongs to:

Emily Warrick

StayWell

StayWell

Cette publication est disponible en français.

The terms he and she have been used throughout the manual to ensure representation of both genders and to correspond to any photos within a particular section.

Illustrations by Jackie Wald
Composition by Embassy Graphics
Printing/binding by Printcrafters Inc.

Printed in Canada by:
The StayWell Health Company Ltd.
2 Quebec Street, Suite 107, Guelph ON N1H 2T3
A division of
StayWell
780 Township Line Road, Yardley, PA 19067-4200 USA

ISBN 13: 978-1-58480-349-2
ISBN 10: 1-58480-349-5

07 08 09 10 / 5 4 3 2

Contents

Acknowledgements

Over the past 50 years, The Canadian Red Cross First Aid Programs have developed and grown. Each time the program undergoes a revision, it starts with a foundation of the great work completed in the previous revision. The last major revision of the First Aid Program was a result of a joint effort between the American Red Cross Society and Mosby-Year Book, Inc. in the early 1990's. We would like to recognize everyone who worked on the programs and products before us.

This revision is dedicated to the memory of Karen Shank, who helped lay the foundation for managing this project.

This project was completed because of the creative vision, ongoing support and dedication of the team at our publishing partner StayWell, the Project Executive Sponsor: Yvan Chalifour, National Director, Injury Prevention, Project Sponsor: Rick Caissie, National Manager First Aid, Project Manager: Cathy Forner, National Project Management Officer, Injury Prevention; and ECC Canada Liaison and Technical Advisor: Tracey Braun, National First Aid Coordinator.

The **Primary Project Team** was responsible for providing the overall leadership, dedication and direction for the project and was made up of: Kelly Ducharme, National Marketing and Promotions Officer; Colleen Lavender, National Marketing and Promotions Officer; Laura McNamara, First Aid Injury Prevention Advisor, Atlantic Zone; Tannis Nostedt, First Aid Program Advisor, Western Zone; Elizabeth Ramlogan, First Aid Services, Program Advisor, Ontario Zone; Eric Ritterrath, National Coordinator, Publications; Sylvie Santerre, Senior Coordinator, Injury Prevention Services, Quebec Zone; Janel Swain, National Project Technical Advisor; and Carolyn Tees, National Marketing and Business Development Officer.

The Canadian Red Cross **National Medical Advisory Team** reviewed the content of the program and was made up of: Brendan J. Hughes MD, CCFP; Andrew MacPherson BSc, MD, CCFP-EM, Chief, Department of Emergency Medicine, Vancouver Island Health Authority, Victoria; and Ernest Prégent MD CCFP(em) CSPQ, FCCFP

External review, guidance, and endorsement of the program content was thanks to: Maureen Shaw, Industrial Accident Prevention Association (IAPA) and Michael Eddy, Canadian Association of Fire Chiefs; Grant Slessor, Dr. Glen Bergeron, PhD, CAT(C), John Boulay, CAT(C), and Ben Trunzo, CAT(C), Canadian Athletic Therapists Association (CATA); Jill Skinner, Canadian Medical Association (CMA); and Peter O'Neil, Smart Risk.

 The Canadian Athletic Therapists Association was pleased to review Chapter 9, Head and Spine Injuries, of this manual.

 The Canadian Medical Association is pleased to support the important work of the Canadian Red Cross in developing this *First Aid and CPR Manual*.

There was excellent market research which guided the project's direction and vision. We would like to thank the many Authorized Providers, Instructor Trainers, and Instructors who participated in the market research. Their input and guidance helped shaped the new look of our programs and products. The **Marketing Project Team** was responsible for marketing expertise and direction for the project and was provided by: Francoise Filteau, Senior Coordinator, Injury Prevention Services, Quebec Zone; Sue Phillips, Director First Aid and Water Safety, Western Zone; and Joan Savoie, Program Representative, Ontario Zone. A Marketing Advisory Panel supported the work of the Marketing Team and we would like to thank the 25 Authorized Providers, Instructors and Instructor Trainers from across Canada that provided their thoughts, advice and direction.

Pupil Training Committee Members - Nolan Baggett, Newfoundland and Labrador; Frédérick Beauchamp, Quebec; Patrick Boucher, Ontario; Troy Conrod, British Columbia; Jan Kirkpatrick, Alberta; Laura MacNeil, Ontario; Tammy Reddekopp, Saskatchewan; Maude St-Onge, Quebec and Mary Wilson, Ontario

Reviewers and Contributors - Alberta – Christie Boyd, Allison Burtnak, Kim Gunn, **British Columbia** – Diana Ferguson, **Manitoba** - Rob Chin, Darryl Toews, Marc Watt, **Ontario** - Peter Alexandrou, Lesley Andrews, Dana Banke, Jo-Anne Brenner, Jason Brinson, Doug Hannum, Jeff Horseman, Mike Nemeth, Butch Snider, **Prince Edward Island** - Garth MacKenzie, **Quebec** – Johane Lafleur, Janet Steinman, **Newfoundland** – Jerry Peach, **Nova Scotia** - Ismael Aquino, Kevin Fitch, John MacKay, Kim Mundle, Christie Swain, Ross Swain, **Saskatchewan** - Lyle Karasiuk, Barry Salmond, **Southern Interior of BC, NWT, Nunavut and Yukon** - Clara Reinhardt

We would also like to express our appreciation to the Ottawa Branch staff and Instructors who graciously agreed to pilot the new programs while they were still being developed.

The Fundamental Principles of the International Red Cross and Red Crescent Movement

Humanity

The International Red Cross and Red Crescent Movement, born of a desire to bring assistance without discrimination to the wounded on the battlefield, endeavours, in its international and national capacity, to prevent and alleviate human suffering wherever it may be found. Its purpose is to protect life and health and ensure respect for the human being. It promotes mutual understanding, friendship, cooperation, and lasting peace amongst all peoples.

Impartiality

It makes no discrimination as to nationality, race, religious beliefs, class, or political opinions. It endeavours to relieve the suffering of individuals, being guided solely by their needs, and to give priority to the most urgent cases of distress.

Neutrality

In order to continue to enjoy the confidence of all, the Movement may not take sides in hostilities or engage at any time in controversies of a political, racial, religious, or ideological nature.

Independence

The Movement is independent. The National Societies, while auxiliaries in the humanitarian services of their governments and subject to the laws of their respective countries, must always maintain their autonomy so that they may be able at all times to act in accordance with the principles of the Movement.

Voluntary Service

It is a voluntary relief movement not prompted in any manner by desire for gain.

Unity

There can be only one Red Cross or one Red Crescent Society in any one country. It must be open to all. It must carry on its humanitarian work throughout its territory.

Universality

The International Red Cross and Red Crescent Movement, in which all Societies have equal status and share equal responsibilities and duties in helping each other, is worldwide.

The Fundamental Principles were proclaimed by the XXth International Conference of the Red Cross, Vienna, 1965. This is the revised text contained in the Statutes of the International Red Cross and the Red Crescent Movement, adopted by the XXVth International Conference of the Red Cross, Geneva, 1986.

In keeping with the Fundamental Principles of the Red Cross, the Society is committed to Social Justice in the elimination of Society structures and actions that oppress, exclude, limit, or discriminate on the basis of race, gender, ethnicity, financial ability, sexual orientation, religion, disability, or age.

The Canadian Red Cross Society

Founded 1896

Incorporated 1909

The red cross emblem and designation "Red Cross" are reserved in Canada by law for the exclusive use of The Canadian Red Cross Society and for the medical units of the armed forces by the Geneva Conventions Act, R.S.C., 1985, c. G-3.

The programs of The Canadian Red Cross Society are made possible by the voluntary services and financial support of the Canadian people.

LOCAL EMERGENCY NUMBERS:

EMS _____

Fire _____

Ambulance _____

Police _____

Poison Control Centre _____

The Red Cross

The Red Cross

The year is 1859. You are a soldier in the French army, and you have been severely wounded. As blood spurts out from a bullet hole in your thigh, you collapse onto the battlefield. You assume that you will die. Later, however, you find yourself confused but alive, lying next to an enemy soldier from the Austrian army. You are no longer on the battlefield, and strangers are tending to the wounds of yourself, your comrades, and your enemies. You are too grateful to be alive to think about war any longer.

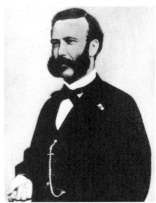

Figure 1.1 Henry Dunant.

HENRY DUNANT – The Red Cross Founder

- In June 1859, Henry Dunant (Figure 1.1) saw an unforgettable scene: 40,000 dead and wounded soldiers left on the field after the Battle of Solferino in Italy.

- Dunant organized local villagers into first aid teams to help as many of the wounded as possible, saving thousands of lives.

NOTE:

In December of 2005, the International Red Cross and Red Crescent Movement welcomed the decision to create an additional emblem alongside the red cross and red crescent, the red crystal.

- To prevent this horror from happening again, he decided to create a neutral organization to care for wounded soldiers and prisoners—an organization that would be respected and protected by both sides in any conflict. The result was the Red Cross.

- Dunant spent the rest of his life trying to reduce the suffering caused by war. He lobbied governments, organized Red Cross Societies in different countries, and spoke to the public.

- Today, the symbol chosen for the Red Cross is recognized around the world: a red cross on a white background.

- In 1901, Dunant won the first Nobel Peace Prize. By founding the International Red Cross and Red Crescent Movement, he saved the lives of millions of people over the years.

THE RED CROSS – Fundamental Principles

There are Red Cross or Red Crescent Societies in over 180 countries around the world.

In every country, our programs and activities are guided by seven Fundamental Principles. The Tanzanian Red Cross has created a short, simple version of these principles:

Humanity: We serve people, but not systems.

Impartiality: We care for the victims and the aggressors alike.

Neutrality: We take initiatives, but never take sides.

Independence: We bow to needs, but not rulers.

Voluntary Service: We work around the clock, but never for personal gain.

Unity: We have many talents, but a single idea.

Universality: We respect nations, but our work knows no bounds.

Essentially, we provide help to people in need, whatever their race, political beliefs, religion, social status, or culture.

WHO WE ARE – The Canadian Red Cross

 Our Mission

The Canadian Red Cross mission is to improve the lives of vulnerable people by mobilizing the power of humanity in Canada and around the world.

 Our Vision

The Canadian Red Cross is the leading humanitarian organization through which people voluntarily demonstrate their caring for others in need.

 Our Values

Our actions and decisions are based on:

• humanitarian values;

• respect, dignity, and care for one another within and outside Red Cross; and

• integrity, accountability, effectiveness, and transparency.

HOW WE HELP

 Disaster Services

Canadian Red Cross helps people affected by emergencies and disasters. We work with governments and with other humanitarian organizations to meet people's basic needs. We provide food, clothing, shelter, first aid, and emotional support. When families have been separated by disasters, we help bring them back together.

 International Programs

Canadian Red Cross works in other countries to help people who have been affected by wars and natural disasters. We bring urgently needed supplies, reunite families, and help rebuild communities. Each year, we send about 100 professional relief workers on overseas missions.

 First Aid Programs

The Canadian Red Cross First Aid Program has been training Canadians in first aid for more than 50 years. Our courses give people the knowledge and skills to deal with emergency situations and to prevent injuries from happening.

 Water Safety Services

Thanks to the work of Water Safety Services, more than 27 million Canadians have learned how to swim and safely enjoy water activities since 1946. Canadian Red Cross also offers an On Board program that gives Canadians everything they need to know to operate pleasure boats safely and to pass the test for their Pleasure Craft Operator Card.

 RespectEd: Violence and Abuse Prevention

Since 1984, this award-winning program has helped more than one million Canadian youth and adults understand abuse, harassment, and interpersonal violence issues.

 Homecare Services

These in-home community services help the frail and elderly, children at risk, people with disabilities, and palliative patients live as independently as possible. Canadian Red Cross has provided these services for more than 70 years.

Preparing to Respond

Preparing to Respond

You are the first to arrive at the scene of a motor vehicle collision. There are two people involved. A woman is sitting by the side of the road with a large cut in her leg, which is bleeding severely. A man is lying on the ground moaning and coughing.

First aid is the immediate care that you give to a sick or injured person until more advanced care can be obtained.

LEVELS OF FIRST AID TRAINING

There are different levels of first aid training:

Emergency first aid deals with life-threatening emergencies. It focusses on airway, breathing, and circulation emergencies.

Standard first aid deals with life-threatening emergencies and with emergencies that could lead to life-threatening situations if they are not treated. It focusses on:

- Airway, breathing, and circulation emergencies
- Injuries to bones, muscles, and joints
- Head and spine injuries
- Sudden medical emergencies
- Wounds
- Poisons
- Heat-related and cold-related emergencies

THE FIRST AIDER'S ROLE

Your role includes three basic steps:

1. Recognize the emergency.

2. Call emergency medical services (EMS)/9-1-1.

3. Act according to your skills, knowledge, and comfort level.

RECOGNIZING EMERGENCIES

The first step in dealing with an emergency is to recognize it:

- A **medical emergency** is an illness or condition that needs immediate medical attention. For example, a heart attack is a medical emergency.

- An **injury** is some kind of damage to the body caused by an external force. This damage can include broken bones, wounds, and burns. The most common causes of injuries include motor vehicle collisions, falls, poisoning, and drowning. Some injuries are serious enough to be considered emergencies. If you're not sure, call EMS/9-1-1 and let the professionals decide.

PREPARE! STAY SAFE! SURVIVE!

- **Prepare!** includes everything you do before you start an activity, including taking a first aid or cardiopulmonary resuscitation (CPR) course.

- **Stay Safe!** includes everything you do during the activity, such as wearing safety gear.

> **REMEMBER:**
>
> *Injuries are not accidents. Injuries are predictable and preventable.*
> *Planning for safety is the best way to prevent injuries.*
> *Good First Aiders keep safe and make wise choices. They help teach friends and family about making wise choices as well.*

- **Survive!** includes actions you take to ensure the safety and the survival of yourself and others, such as reporting hazards at your workplace or providing first aid in an emergency.

DECIDE TO ACT

Many lives are saved because people like you get involved. Every year many bystanders in Canada recognize and respond to emergencies. Some phone for help, some comfort the ill or injured person or family members, some give first aid, and some help keep order at the emergency scene.

One of the simplest and most important ways of providing first aid is to call for help (EMS/9-1-1). By making this call, you'll make sure that highly trained medical professionals arrive to care for the ill or injured person (Figure 2.1).

Sometimes people don't want to get involved in an emergency for various reasons. The five most common concerns are:

Other people at the scene: If there are other people at the scene, it's easy to think that they can take care of the emergency without your help. However, you should never assume that someone is providing first aid just because you see a lot of people. And remember that there are many important jobs that you can do. You can help control the crowd, call EMS/9-1-1, get supplies, or comfort the ill or injured person.

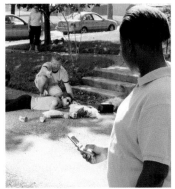

Figure 2.1 Calling EMS/9-1-1.

The ill or injured person: You may not feel comfortable treating people if they are behaving oddly, if they are much older or younger than you, or if they are of a different race or gender. Remember, whoever they are, they need help.

Unpleasant injuries or illnesses: You may feel upset or sick when you see blood, vomit, broken bones, or other injuries. If this happens, take a few deep breaths to help calm yourself before you deal with the situation.

Catching a disease: You might have a concern that you could catch something from the injured person. There are many ways to reduce the risks, and we'll discuss them in this chapter. If you take simple precautions while performing basic first aid, they can limit the possibility of catching a serious disease.

Doing something wrong: You might be afraid of getting sued if you make a mistake. As long as you act reasonably and carefully, you don't need to worry. All provinces and territories have laws to protect bystanders who give emergency help. Just use common sense and don't try to do something that you're not trained to do. Once you start giving first aid, keep providing help until EMS personnel arrive.

Thinking about these things now and mentally preparing yourself for an emergency will help you overcome your fears.

GET CONSENT

Once you decide to act, get the ill or injured person's consent. To get consent, you must tell the person three things:

1. Who you are

2. That you are trained in first aid

3. That you are here to help

If a baby or a child is ill or injured:

• Ask the supervising adult for consent.

• If the baby or child is alone, you can assume you have consent to give first aid.

If the person refuses your help:

• Have someone call EMS/9-1-1. Let them know the person has refused help. The EMS personnel who arrive will deal with the situation.

• Do not try to give help.

• Stay nearby if possible.

> **NOTE:**
> *If the situation is a life-threatening one, the parent or guardian cannot legally refuse to give consent.*

PREPARING FOR EMERGENCIES

By being prepared for emergencies, you can make sure that an ill or injured person gets help as soon as possible. First aid training gives you a plan of action for any emergency and gives you the confidence to act.

After you have learned first aid, stay prepared for emergencies by practising regularly. Think of emergencies that could happen in your home or workplace and rehearse how you would respond. Make sure your family and co-workers know what to do in all types of emergencies. Suggest that they take a first aid course too.

PREPARING FOR EMERGENCIES AT HOME

- Keep important information about you and your family in a handy place. Include your address, everyone's date of birth, health card numbers, medical conditions, allergies, and prescriptions and dosages. List the names and phone numbers of your doctors.

- Keep your medical records up to date.

- Post the numbers for the police, fire department, EMS, and Poison Control Centre near every phone in your home.

- Teach children how to call for help.

- Install smoke and carbon monoxide detectors. Test them regularly.

- Keep a first aid kit handy in your home, car, and workplace.

- Learn and practise first aid skills such as CPR.

- Make sure your house or apartment number is easy to see.

- You should wear a MedicAlert® medical identification product if you have a potentially serious medical condition such as epilepsy, diabetes, heart disease, or allergies.

AFTER AN EMERGENCY

After dealing with an emergency it is often helpful to talk to somebody about the situation. If you are really bothered, you can contact your local crisis intervention line or look in the front of your phone book for information on whom to contact.

As a First Aider you can help others involved in the emergency by talking to them and providing comfort.

PREPARING FOR DISASTERS

Disasters and personal emergencies can and do happen anywhere in Canada.

The key to being prepared is to identify what disasters could happen in your home, workplace, and recreational area.

PREPARING FOR DISASTERS AT HOME

- Talk with your family about the dangers of fire, severe weather, and other emergencies that could happen in your area.

- Pick two meeting places—one near your home to use in case of fire and one outside the neighbourhood to use in case you cannot return home after a disaster.

- Keep family records in a waterproof and fireproof container.

- Have emergency supply kits handy.

- Call Canadian Red Cross for disaster education program information, or visit our Website at www.redcross.ca.

AFTER A DISASTER

- Move people away from unsafe areas.

- Unless you need to call EMS/9-1-1, don't use the telephone.

- If you have been separated from your family, register with the local Red Cross.

- If you have to evacuate your home, wear sturdy shoes and clothing that will keep you comfortable. Take your emergency supplies kit. Lock your home when you leave and use the travel routes that local officials recommend.

To prepare for emergencies and disasters in the workplace, follow your employer's protocol.

INFECTION

An **infection** is a disease caused by germs that invade your body.

For someone to get an infection or infectious disease, four things must happen:

1. Germs must be present in the surrounding environment.

2. The germs must enter the body.

3. Enough germs must be present in the body to cause infection.

4. The individual's natural defences must be weak.

If any one of these are missing, you won't get an infection. For example, germs present on your skin cannot harm you if they cannot enter your body. If you are immune to a particular disease because you have received a vaccination, your immune system will kill the germs in your body that cause the particular disease before you become infected.

Knowing how germs are spread will help you understand how to prevent infection.

▶ How Is an Infection Spread From One Person to Another?

There are four different ways that infections can be spread from one person to another:

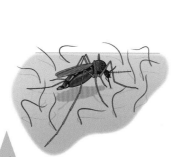

1. Direct contact
— for example, when you touch the blood of someone who is infected.

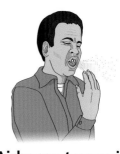

2. Indirect contact
— for example, when you pick up something that an infected person has touched.

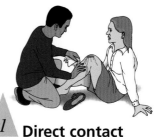

3. Airborne transmission
— for example, when an infected person sneezes, sending germs into the air, and you breathe in those germs.

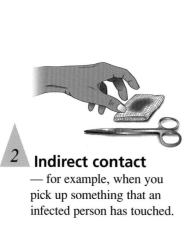

4. Vector transmission
— for example, when a mosquito bites an infected person and then bites you, passing on the germs.

Some infections are spread through only one of these routes. Others may be spread through several routes.

▶ How to Prevent Diseases From Spreading

There are some basic precautions that you can take to stop diseases from spreading:

Type of Precaution	Definition	Example
Personal Precautions	Actions that individuals can take to reduce the risk of spreading disease	Wash your hands frequently and thoroughly. See "hand washing" on page 14. Treat all blood and other body fluids as infectious materials. Cover your mouth and nose when you sneeze. Eat well and get enough exercise and sleep.
Equipment Precautions	Items that protect you from direct contact with contaminated objects	Always use some type of barrier device between you and any material that could be infected. Wear safety glasses, goggles, masks, gloves (choose non-latex or safety gloves), and any other personal protective equipment your workplace specifies. If there is a chance you might get splashed with body fluids, wear safety glasses or a face shield. Use dressings to minimize your contact with blood. **NOTE:** *You must use personal protective equipment in the workplace. However, if you are helping a family member, it is your choice whether you use personal protective equipment.*
Environmental Precautions	The set-up of an area that reduces exposure to germs	Make sure there is proper ventilation in your workplace. Make sure that people don't use the same sink for hygiene and food preparation. Dispose of any contaminated materials immediately. **NOTE:** *Many environmental precautions are the responsibility of the employer, but you can make suggestions if you notice something.*

▶ Hand Washing

Hand washing is an important precaution wherever you are. It helps prevent you from spreading germs that can cause many infectious diseases. Use the following guidelines for washing your hands:

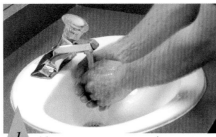

1 Always use warm running water and a mild soap.

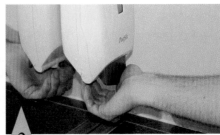

2 Wet your hands and apply a small amount of soap (use liquid soap if possible; you can use an antibacterial soap if you want to, but it isn't necessary), approximately the size of a dime or a quarter.

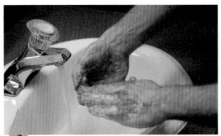

3 Rub your hands together vigorously until you see a soapy lather. Keep rubbing your hands for at least 15 seconds. Make sure you scrub between your fingers, under your fingernails, and around the backs and palms of your hands.

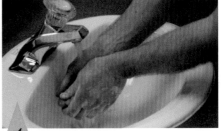

4 Rinse your hands under warm running water. Leave the water running while you dry your hands.

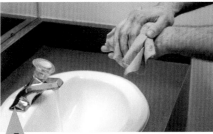

5 Dry your hands with a clean, disposable towel. Be careful not to touch the faucet handles or the towel holder with your clean hands.

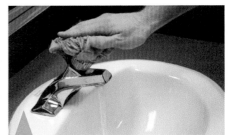

6 Turn the faucet off using the towel as a barrier between your hands and the faucet handle. Throw the used towel into a trash can that is lined with a plastic bag. Trash cans with lids that you can open with a foot pedal are best.

You should wash your hands:

- Before and after contact with an ill or injured person

- After removing gloves

- After helping in an emergency

- When your hands look dirty

- Before eating or drinking

- After handling dirty articles, instruments, or dressings

- Before or after treating wounds

- Before going home from work

> Hand sanitizers and alcohol hand-rubs are appropriate for rapidly decontaminating your hands if they are otherwise clean. They are not a substitute for hand washing if your hands are soiled. When you can see dirt on your hands, you should first wash them with soap and water.

▶ Gloves

When you take off a pair of gloves, make sure that the outside of the glove doesn't touch your skin. Always wash your hands after you take off gloves.

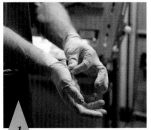

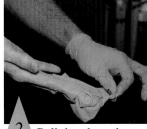

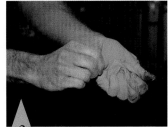

1 Pinch the glove at the wrist, being careful to touch only the glove's outside surface.

2 Pull the glove down and off.

3 Form the glove into a ball and hold it in the other hand. Insert thumb under inside rim of other glove, on palm side; push glove inside out and down onto fingers and over balled glove. Discard gloves appropriately.

> Some people are allergic to latex. For some people, latex causes a mild skin rash. For others, it can cause a life-threatening reaction called anaphylaxis. When you're giving first aid, always check for MedicAlert® medical identification products that will tell you if the person has a serious illness or allergy.

Immunization

Most people have been immunized against common childhood diseases such as measles and mumps (Figure 2.2). Immunization intro- duces a substance into your body that builds up your resistance against the germs that cause a specific disease.

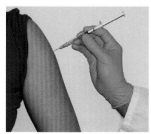

Figure 2.2 Immunization helps prevent illness and disease.

Children usually get immunizations because they are required for school or sports programs. However, not all adults have been immunized. Talk to your doctor or local community health nurse about your immunizations.

If you are planning a trip outside the country, find out well before you plan to travel which immunizations you need for the countries you will visit.

Immunizations not only protect you, they also protect your family, friends, and co-workers.

> Because the risk of disease varies from place to place, this manual can't cover all the hazards that you might face. For specific guidelines on your particular situation, talk to your doctor or call your community public health centre.

The Emergency Medical Services System

The Emergency Medical Services System

While you're driving on a rural road, the car in front of you suddenly goes off the road and rolls into a ditch. You see that the air bag has deployed, and you reach for your cell phone.

THE EMERGENCY MEDICAL SERVICES SYSTEM

The emergency medical services (EMS) system is a network of community resources and personnel organized to give emergency care in cases of injury or sudden illness. It varies from community to community. In many areas you can call 9-1-1, whereas other areas have a different local number. The level of training of the emergency medical personnel may also vary.

WHO IS COMING TO HELP?

There are several different kinds of trained personnel who may respond after you call for help.

First Responders: These include police, firefighters, or job-specific personnel such as athletic trainers or industrial safety personnel (Figure 3.1).

Paramedics: These are highly specialized emergency personnel who can often administer medications, including medications that are given intravenously (through IVs) in some cases. They provide the highest level of pre-hospital care.

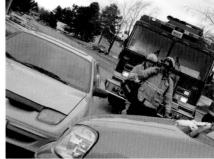

Figure 3.1 A First Responder in action.

WHEN TO CALL EMS/9-1-1

Trust your instincts. If you think that an emergency exists, it probably does. Do not lose time calling friends or family members—call EMS/9-1-1 for professional help immediately. It is better for these professionals to come and find out they are not needed than not come in an emergency when they were needed.

You should call EMS/9-1-1 in cases of:

- Danger to you or to others
- Unconsciousness or an altered level of consciousness
- Difficulty breathing or no signs of breathing
- Persistent chest pain or pressure (lasting longer than 10 minutes)
- Deadly bleeding
- Seizures, severe headache, or slurred speech
- Injuries to the head, neck, or back
- Blood in the vomit, urine, or stool
- Imminent childbirth

In addition to the cases listed above, you should call EMS/9-1-1 if the ill or injured person is involved in or exposed to the following:

- Fire or explosion
- Poisonous gas
- Swift-moving water
- Motor vehicle collision
- Live electrical wires
- A situation where you cannot get to the ill or injured person easily

Contact your local Poison Control Centre for any suspected poisoning.

HOW TO CALL EMS/9-1-1

When you call, the EMS dispatcher who answers will likely ask:

- Where is the emergency?
- What telephone number are you calling from?
- What is your name?
- What has happened?
- How many people are involved and what is their condition?

Don't hang up until the dispatcher tells you to.

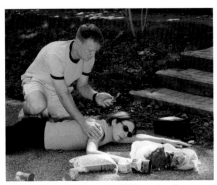

Figure 3.2 Calling EMS/9-1-1 when you are alone.

Sending someone else to call the emergency number is better than calling it yourself because it means that you can stay with the ill or injured person and keep giving first aid. If you are alone with the person, call out loudly for help. If no one comes, get to a phone as quickly as you can to call EMS/9-1-1 (Figure 3.2). As soon as you hang up, return to the person to keep giving help.

If someone else can make the call for you, ask him to come back and tell you what the EMS/9-1-1 dispatcher said. If he has a cell phone, he can stay with you.

MOVING A PERSON BEFORE PROVIDING CARE

NOTE:

If you cannot wait for EMS personnel to arrive and you must move the person, follow the guidelines. ALWAYS ENSURE YOUR OWN SAFETY.

Move an ill or injured person only if:

- The person's position stops you from giving care for a life-threatening injury or illness.

- The ill or injured person is blocking access to someone with a more serious injury or illness.

- The person is likely to drown.

- The scene is becoming unsafe.

REMEMBER:

In any situation, never put yourself in danger. Before you try to move someone, make sure you have whatever supplies you need to do it safely.

Clothes Drag

To move someone who may have a head, neck, or back injury:

1. Hold the person's clothing behind the person's neck.

2. Pull the person to safety.

3. While moving the person, cradle the head with the person's clothes and your hands. Keep the person's head, neck, and back in a straight line as best as you can.

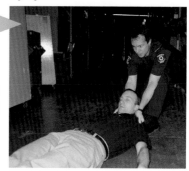

Two-Person Seat Carry

To carry someone who cannot walk and isn't likely to have a head, neck, or back injury:

1. Stand on one side of the person and have another First Aider stand on the other side.

2. Put one arm under the person's thighs and the other across the person's back while the other First Aider does the same thing.

3. Hold the other First Aider's wrists underneath the person's legs and across the person's back. Have the other First Aider hold your wrists.

4. Move the person to safety.

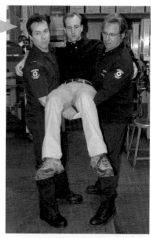

Walking Assist

To move someone who needs help walking to safety:

1. Have the person stand up.

2. Stand on the person's weak or injured side and put his arm across your shoulders. Hold it there with one hand.

3. Support the person with your other hand around the waist.

4. Move the person to safety.

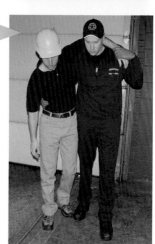

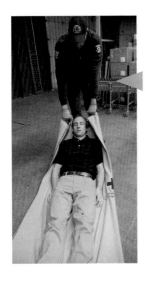

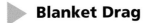 **Blanket Drag**

To move someone in an emergency situation when you don't have a stretcher:

1. Keep the person between you and the blanket.

2. Gather half the blanket and place it against the person's side.

3. Roll the person towards you. Make sure the person's body moves as a unit.

4. Reach over and pull the blanket towards the person so that you can roll the person on top of it.

5. Roll the person back, onto the blanket.

6. Gather the blanket at the head and move the person to safety.

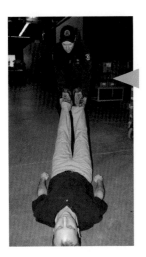

▶ **Foot Drag**

To move someone who cannot otherwise be carried or moved:

1. Firmly grasp the person's ankles and move backwards.

2. Pull the person in a straight line, being careful not to bump the person's head.

▶ Assisting a Near-Drowning Person With a Reaching Assist

To rescue someone who is far out in the water:

1 Call for a lifeguard or other trained person. You need special training to swim out to rescue someone. If you do not have proper training, entering the water to help a person is dangerous. The person may try to hold onto you and is likely to pull you under the water.

To rescue someone who is nearby in the water:

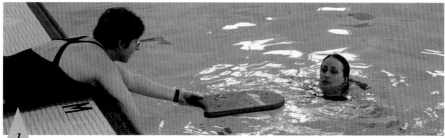

1 Find something that you can hold out to reach the person, such as a pole, oar or paddle, tree branch, shirt, belt, or towel.

Lie down in a safe position. The best is lying down at a 45-degree angle to the side of the dock or pool with your legs spread out to keep you stable. Firmly brace yourself so that you won't get pulled into the water. If you can't lie down, crouch or bend on one knee, staying as far from the water's edge as you can.

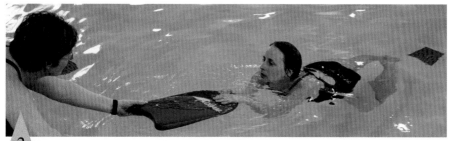

2 Hold out your reaching assist for the person to grab.

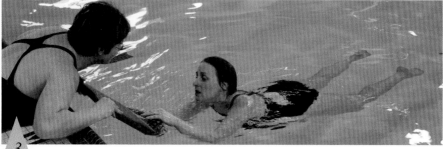

3 Pull the reaching assist back in and then move to the edge of the water to secure the person.

NOTES:

Check, Call, Care

Check, Call, Care

At the local playground, a three-year-old boy has fallen from the top of a slide and is lying on the ground, screaming in pain. You are one of three people trained in first aid to come to the scene and offer help.

PRIMARY SURVEY

 Check

Once you recognize an emergency, take time to look around and do the following before you begin to help:

Check the Scene

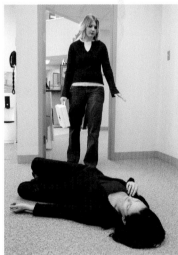

- Is it safe (Figure 4.1)? *Look* for things such as glass, hostile bystanders, or oncoming cars; *listen* for things such as alarms or escaping gas; and *smell* for things such as gas or smoke.

- What happened? How did it happen?

- How many ill or injured people are there?

- Is there someone to help me?

- Is there someone who looks to be unconscious?

Figure 4.1 Check the scene for safety.

Preventing Disease Transmission

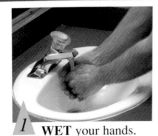

1 **WET** your hands.

2 Apply a small amount of **SOAP**, about the size of a dime or a quarter.

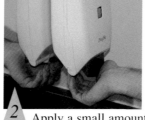

3 Make sure you **SCRUB** between your fingers, under your fingernails, and around the backs and palms of your hands.

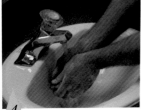

4 **RINSE** your hands under warm running water. Leave the water running while you dry your hands.

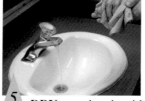

5 **DRY** your hands with a clean, disposable towel. Be careful not to touch the faucet handles or the towel holder with your clean hands.

6 Turn the faucet off using the towel as a **BARRIER** between your hands and the faucet handle.

Canadian Red Cross   1-877-356-3226 | www.redcross.ca

Preventing Disease Transmission

PERSONAL PROTECTIVE EQUIPMENT

Always use some type of barrier device between you and possible infected material.

- Choose non-latex or safety gloves

- Goggles

- Masks

- Safety glasses

- Workplace specific safety equipment

ENVIRONMENTAL PRECAUTIONS

- Proper ventilation in your workplace

- Separate sinks for hygiene and food preparation

 Canadian Red Cross   1-877-356-3226 | www.redcross.ca

When More Than One Person Is Ill or Injured

If you are ever in a situation where there are several ill or injured people, the general principle is to do what is best for the most people. This is called *triage.*

As an example, if someone has minor bleeding and another person has more deadly bleeding, you should help the person with deadly bleeding because EMS personnel will arrive before the minor bleeding becomes serious. Deadly bleeding is life-threatening **right now.** If you have to decide who needs your help most urgently, trust your own judgment to do what is best for the most people.

Check the Person

1. If it is safe to do so, check the person (Figure 4.2):

    - Ask the person "Are you okay?" Use the person's name if you know it.

    - Tap the person on the shoulder.

If there is no response, call EMS/9-1-1.

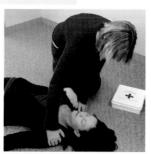
Figure 4.2 Check the person.

An ill or injured person may have an altered level of consciousness. They may be unresponsive to your voice or confused about time and place.

2. Does she want your help? Tell her:

    - Who you are

    - That you are trained in first aid

    - That you are here to help

If someone is unconscious or can't answer because of the illness or injury, you can assume you have consent to give first aid.

Never risk your own safety. Leave dangerous situations for EMS personnel.

▶ Call

- If the person does not respond, have someone call EMS/9-1-1(Figure 4.3).

- If you are alone:
    - ▶ For an adult, call EMS/9-1-1 yourself and return to giving care (ex. CPR).
    - ▶ For a child or baby, do five cycles (2 minutes) of CPR, if necessary, then make the call and return to giving care.

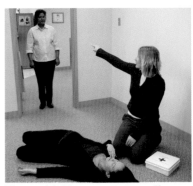

Figure 4.3 Have someone call EMS/9-1-1.

> **REMEMBER:**
>
> *Before you give care, you should take personal precautions. Wear gloves and use a barrier device.*

▶ Care

The ABCs: Airway, Breathing, and Circulation

A = Check the Airway

Your first job is to make sure the person has an open airway. The airway is the pathway from the mouth and nose to the lungs. If it is closed or obstructed, air cannot get in, making it impossible to breathe. Anyone who can speak or cry has an open airway.

If the person is unconscious, you must make sure the airway is open. To do this, tilt the head back and lift the chin (Figure 4.4). This action moves the tongue away from the back of the throat and lets air reach the lungs.

Figure 4.4 Open the airway.

You'll learn more about dealing with airway emergencies in Chapter 5.

B = Check Breathing

Next, check for breathing. Someone who can speak or cry is breathing.

Check for normal breathing for no more than 10 seconds (Figure 4.5). *Look* at an unconscious person carefully for signs of normal

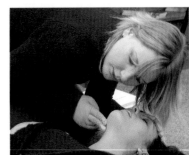

Figure 4.5 Check for normal breathing.

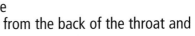

breathing. The chest should rise and fall. You must also *listen* and *feel* for normal breathing. Put your face close so you can hear and feel air coming out the nose and mouth while you watch the chest rising and falling.

C = Check Circulation

Checking circulation means looking for deadly bleeding and signs of shock (Figure 4.6). Quickly look at the person from head to toe. Deadly bleeding must be controlled as soon as possible. You will learn how to do this in Chapter 6.

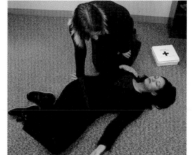

Figure 4.6 Check circulation.

Also, if the person is breathing normally (more than an occasional gasp), it means that the heart is beating. However, if the person is not breathing normally, the heart may soon stop, so you should start compressions. You will learn how to do this in Chapter 7.

NOTE: If the person is not breathing normally, this must be treated before checking circulation.

NOTE: If there is someone there to help, they can treat deadly bleeding or treat for shock while you treat other life-threatening emergencies.

▶ Shock

NOTE: Treat for shock if ABCs are okay.

Shock happens when the vital organs do not get enough oxygen-rich blood for any reason. It is a very common condition that can affect the people involved in an emergency situation. Treat shock very seriously: it can be fatal.

Bystanders and First Aiders can be affected by emotional shock. Although this condition is not fatal, you should watch for it and treat it if it occurs.

Causes of Shock

You should be on the lookout for shock with any injury, sudden illness, or involvement in a serious incident.

It is often caused by:

- Too much blood loss
- Extensive burns
- Too much fluid loss—because of diarrhea and vomiting, for example, especially in children
- A weak heart
- Infection
- Emotion due to the impact of an event

---

breathing. The chest should rise and fall. You must also *listen* and *feel* for normal breathing. Put your face close so you can hear and feel air coming out the nose and mouth while you watch the chest rising and falling.

C = Check Circulation

Checking circulation means looking for deadly bleeding and signs of shock (Figure 4.6). Quickly look at the person from head to toe. Deadly bleeding must be controlled as soon as possible. You will learn how to do this in Chapter 6.

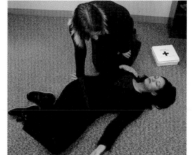

Figure 4.6 Check circulation.

Also, if the person is breathing normally (more than an occasional gasp), it means that the heart is beating. However, if the person is not breathing normally, the heart may soon stop, so you should start compressions. You will learn how to do this in Chapter 7.

NOTE: *If the person is not breathing normally, this must be treated before checking circulation.*

NOTE: *If there is someone there to help, they can treat deadly bleeding or treat for shock while you treat other life-threatening emergencies.*

▶ Shock

NOTE: *Treat for shock if ABCs are okay.*

Shock happens when the vital organs do not get enough oxygen-rich blood for any reason. It is a very common condition that can affect the people involved in an emergency situation. Treat shock very seriously: it can be fatal.

Bystanders and First Aiders can be affected by emotional shock. Although this condition is not fatal, you should watch for it and treat it if it occurs.

Causes of Shock

You should be on the lookout for shock with any injury, sudden illness, or involvement in a serious incident.

It is often caused by:

- Too much blood loss
- Extensive burns
- Too much fluid loss—because of diarrhea and vomiting, for example, especially in children
- A weak heart
- Infection
- Emotion due to the impact of an event

Signs and Symptoms of Shock

- Anxiety
- Skin that is paler than normal
- Confusion
- Rapid breathing
- Nausea and vomiting

- Cold, clammy skin
- Weakness
- Excessive thirst
- Drowsiness or loss of consciousness

 First Aid for Shock

While you are waiting for EMS personnel to arrive:

 1 Care for the cause of the shock.

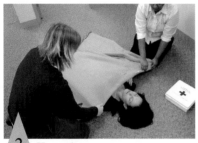

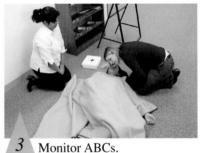

2 Keep the person warm.

3 Monitor ABCs.

 4 Have the person rest.

 5 Give comfort and reassurance.

NOTE:

Only move to a secondary survey if ABCs are okay.

SECONDARY SURVEY

If the person's ABCs are present, you need to find out what else may be wrong. To do this, you should do a secondary survey of the person to look for injuries that are not life-threatening at this point in time. There are three parts to this:

1. Ask **questions.** Interview the person (if she is conscious) and other people at the scene to get more information.

2. Check **vital signs.** Check for consciousness, breathing, and skin colour and temperature.

    Skin that is paler than usual and lips that are bluish indicate problems with circulation.

3. Check the person for injuries from **head to toe.**

If you can, write down what you find during the secondary survey or have someone else write it down or help you remember. When EMS personnel arrive, give them the notes or tell them what you learned.

NOTE:

Always complete the secondary survey before treating any non-life-threatening injuries. If the person has minor bleeding, have him or her hold a clean cloth or gauze pad over the wound while you complete the survey.

▶ **Ask Questions**

Get more information by asking the SAMPLE questions:

S = Signs and symptoms

Are there any cuts or bruises? How do you feel? Is there any pain?

A = Allergies

Are you allergic to anything?

M = Medications

Do you take any medicine? What is it for?

P = Past medical history

Do you have any medical conditions such as heart disease or another illness? Has this happened before?

L = Last meal

When did you last eat? What did you eat?

E = Events leading up to the emergency

What happened?

> *Signs* are signals of illness or injury that a First Aider can see, hear, or feel when checking the ill or injured person.
>
> *Symptoms* are things the ill or injured person says that he or she feels.

▶ **Check Vital Signs**

Level of consciousness Is the person awake or sleepy? Does the person seem confused? Is the person responsive?

Breathing Listen for sounds. Is the breathing fast or slow, shallow or deep? Is breathing painful for the person?

Skin Is it dry or wet? Is it an unusual colour or temperature?

Head-to-Toe Check

The goal of a head-to-toe check is to look carefully and systematically for injuries that aren't life-threatening.

Remember:

- Be careful not to cause further injury!

- Start by telling the person what you are going to do and ask the person to stay still.

- Avoid touching any painful areas or having the person move any area that hurts.

- Watch the person's expression.

- Look for a MedicAlert® medical identification product. This may tell you what might be wrong, whom to call for help, and what care to give.

A MedicAlert® medical identification product indicates that the person wearing it has a particular medical condition. In the event of an emergency or non-critical medical situation, MedicAlert® lets emergency responders and healthcare providers immediately access a member's medical record, anytime and from anywhere in the world. These products include bracelets, necklaces, watch straps, wallet cards, and anklets.

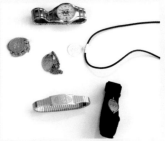

Hands-Off Check

If the person is conscious and able to answer questions, do a hands-off check.

As you do this check keep watching the person's level of consciousness, breathing, and skin colour. If any problems develop, *stop* whatever you are doing and give first aid *immediately*.

2 Look at all areas of the body that are not covered by clothing for discoloration (bruises) or deformities (odd shapes).

1 Start by telling the person what you are going to do and ask the person to stay still.

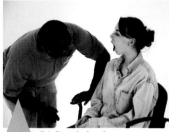

4 Ask the person to move each body part one at a time, beginning with the head, to see if anything hurts.

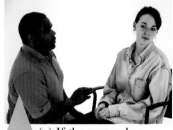

3 Look at the appearance of the skin and check its temperature with the back of your hand. A person with a breathing problem may have a face that is flushed or paler than normal. Cool, moist skin that is paler than normal often indicates shock. For privacy reasons, don't remove any articles of clothing from the person unless the clothing makes first aid difficult.

(a) If the person has neck pain, do not move the neck. If there is no neck pain, ask if the person can slowly move his or her head from side to side.

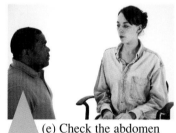

(b) Look in the ears, nose, and mouth for blood or fluids.

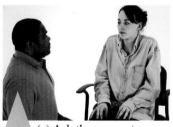

(c) Ask the person to shrug his or her shoulders. Ask if there is any pain or discomfort.

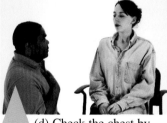

(d) Check the chest by asking the person to take a deep breath and then blow the air out.

(e) Check the abdomen by asking the person to push the stomach out and then pull it in.

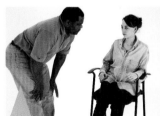

(f) Check the hips by asking the person to move the hips slightly.

- If there is no pain in the hips, ask the person to wiggle the toes.
- If there is no pain in the toes, ask the person to move the ankles.
- If there is no pain in the ankles, ask the person to bend the knees.

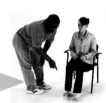

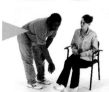

(g) Check the hands by asking the person to wiggle the fingers.

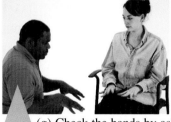

- If there is no pain in the fingers, ask the person to move the wrists.

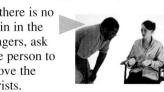

- If there is no pain in the wrists, ask the person to move the elbows.

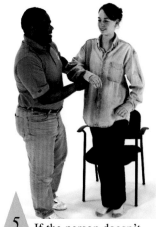

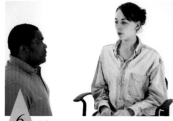

 5 If the person doesn't complain of any pain and doesn't have any tender areas or signs of injury, ask the person to rest for a few minutes in a comfortable position. Check the vital signs and monitor the ABCs. If you see no problem, help the person to stand up slowly when he or she is ready.

6 If the person has pain or dizziness or cannot move a body part, check the ABCs again. Have the person rest, help keep the body temperature normal, and give reassurance. If you find any injuries, provide first aid as needed and decide whether you need to call EMS/9-1-1.

▶ Hands-On Check

You may need to do a hands-on check to assess whether further first aid is required. Do not perform a hands-on check unless you can be sure that the airway will not be compromised.

This check is mainly for an unconscious person who cannot tell you what is wrong. A conscious person will probably not like being touched. If the person is conscious, you may need to do a hands-on check at the site of the injury, but the entire check is not always necessary.

As you do this examination, keep watching the person's level of consciousness, breathing, and skin (vital signs). If any problems develop, *stop* whatever you are doing and give first aid *immediately*.

> **NOTE:**
> *Remember to wear your gloves when performing the hands-on check.*

Chapter 4

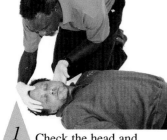

1 Check the head and neck. Look and feel for any abnormalities such as bumps, soft spots, or bleeding. Do not push on soft spots—they may be fractures of the skull.

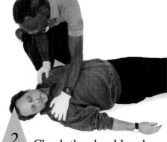

2 Check the shoulders by looking and feeling for any bumps or bone deformities.

NOTE:

Be careful not to reach underneath someone because there could be glass or other objects that could hurt you. Look around and under the body for any signs of blood or fluids.

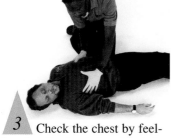

3 Check the chest by feeling the ribs for deformity. Ask the person to take a deep breath; both sides of the rib cage should expand at the same time. If any part of the ribs moves differently from the rest when the person breathes in or out, call EMS/9-1-1.

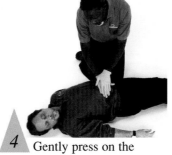

4 Gently press on the abdomen to see if it is hard.

- The abdomen should feel soft to the touch. If the abdomen is painful or hard to the touch, you may have to move clothing and check for bruising.

- Do not poke or push on a hard, painful, or bruised abdomen.

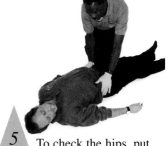

5 To check the hips, put your hands on both sides of the pelvis and push down on the hips and then in on the sides. The hip bones should move together. Do not push or pull if the person shows any signs of discomfort.

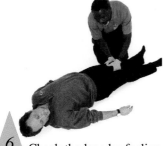

6 Check the legs by feeling for any deformity in the bones or any swelling.

7 Check the arms by feeling for any deformity in the bones or any swelling.

Complete all the steps of your secondary survey and then treat any injuries you have found. Treatment for various injuries is explained in the following chapters.

CONTINUAL CARE

After your secondary survey it is important to keep the person comfortable and monitor the ABCs continually until EMS personnel arrive.

 ## Recovery Position

Once you've checked the ABCs and you have completed your secondary survey, you should move an unconscious person into the *recovery position* if:

1. the airway is open;

2. the person is breathing;

3. there is no deadly bleeding; and

4. you don't suspect there is a neck or back injury.

The recovery position keeps the airway open and allows any blood or vomit to drain from the mouth, which is why it's also called the *drainage position.*

If you have to leave the person alone, you should put her in the recovery position. To move someone into the recovery position if the person is on her back:

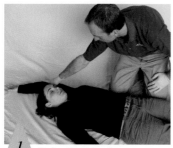

1 Raise the arm closest to you.

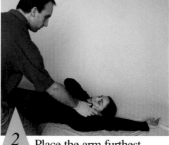

2 Place the arm furthest from you across the person's chest with the palm against the cheek.

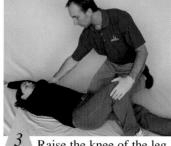

3 Raise the knee of the leg further away from you.

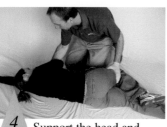

4 Support the head and neck with one hand as you pull the person towards you with your other hand on the raised leg close to the knee. Position the person on his or her side with knee out in front and hip at right angle to prevent the person from rolling onto his or her face.

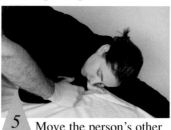

5 Move the person's other arm into a position of comfort in front of the body.

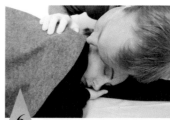

6 Treat for shock and monitor vital signs.

▶ Should You Drive an Ill or Injured Person to Hospital?

Never try to drive an ill or injured person anywhere yourself if the condition is life-threatening or if it might become life-threatening, such as chest pain, which may lead to cardiac arrest. Instead, call EMS/9-1-1 and wait for help. A car or boat trip may make things worse.

If the person is a friend or family member, and if you are sure the person's injuries are minor, you may decide to take them to a hospital, doctor's office or nursing station yourself. Take someone else with you to help keep the person comfortable and to watch for any changes in their condition.

Never let an ill or injured person drive alone to get help. If the person's condition gets worse, it could be unsafe to drive.

SUMMARY:

▶ Check:

- Check the scene.
- Check the person.

▶ Call:

- Call EMS/9-1-1.

▶ Care:

- Deal with life-threatening conditions (ABCs).

▶ Secondary Survey:

- Perform a secondary survey and treat any non-life-threatening injuries.

▶ Continual Care:

- Keep the person comfortable and monitor vital signs.

NOTES:

Airway
Emergencies

Airway Emergencies

At a family barbeque, your three-year-old nephew is finishing a hot dog as he runs over to join his older cousins, who are playing on a swing set. He starts to cough, so you go over to help. When you get close, he stops coughing, grabs his throat, and starts to turn blue.

The airway is the passage that connects the nose and mouth with the lungs. If anything blocks the airway (Figure 5.1), the person chokes and cannot get enough oxygen. This is a life-threatening emergency, and you must give first aid to remove whatever is blocking the airway.

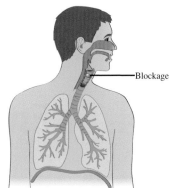

Figure 5.1 A blockage in the airway.

MILD CHOKING

Coughing may indicate a mild airway obstruction. Coughing is a natural way to clear the airway, and it is a sign that the person is still getting enough air. Encourage the person to keep coughing and stay close by in case you need to help. An object may become more firmly stuck in the airway, stopping the person from breathing.

SEVERE CHOKING

Severe choking happens when a foreign object or swelling blocks the airway completely. The object may get stuck at any point in the airway from the throat to the lungs. This is a severe airway obstruction.

► Causes of Choking

- Trying to swallow large pieces of food
- Drinking too much alcohol before or during meals because alcohol affects muscle reflexes
- Eating while talking, walking, running, or playing

► Preventing Choking

In adults:

- Chew food well before swallowing.
- Eat slowly and calmly.
- Do not talk, laugh, walk, or do other kinds of physical activitiy with food in your mouth.
- Do not drink too much alcohol before or during meals.

In children:

- Do not let young children move around with food in their hands or mouth. Constantly watch children when they are eating.
- Feed babies or young children appropriate soft foods in small pieces.
- Make sure there are no small objects nearby that babies or young children might put in their mouth.
- Keep young children away from balloons, which can burst into small pieces that can be easily inhaled.

► Signs and Symptoms of Severe Choking

- Inability to breathe
- Inability to speak
- Inability to cough
- Change in face colour (a face that is bluish or paler than normal)
- Look of panic with wide eyes
- One or both hands clutching the throat (Figure 5.2)

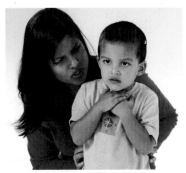

Figure 5.2 The universal sign for choking.

First Aid

Conscious Choking

Adult or Child

Check:

- Check the scene for danger.
- If it is safe to do so, check the person.

Call:

- Shout for help.

Care:

> **NOTE:**
>
> *To determine if choking is mild or severe, ask "Are you choking?" If the person can speak, cough, or breathe, it is mild choking.*

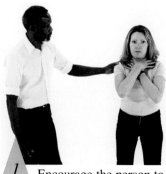

1 Encourage the person to continue coughing and do not interfere. The obstruction might clear itself.

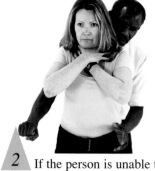

2 If the person is unable to speak or breathe or has wheezing breathing, it is severe choking. Stand (or kneel for a small child) behind the person and wrap both arms around the abdomen.

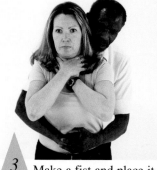

3 Make a fist and place it just above the belly button.

- Place your other hand over the fist and pull sharply in and up.
- Continue until the object comes out or the person becomes unconscious.

If the object comes out:

Secondary Survey:

Perform a secondary survey and treat any non-life-threatening injuries.

Continual Care:

Provide continual care.

If the person becomes unconscious:

Support the person to the ground, protecting the head, and place the person on her back. Call EMS/9-1-1 and follow the steps for unconscious choking.

 For a Larger or Pregnant Person:

If someone is too large for you to wrap your arms around to give abdominal thrusts, or if a woman is obviously pregnant, give chest thrusts:

1. Stand behind the person and wrap both arms around the chest just under the armpits.

2. Make a fist and place the thumb side in the middle of the person's chest.

3. Place your other hand over your fist and pull straight back towards you. If the first couple of thrusts aren't effective, pull more sharply and deeply.

4. Continue until the object comes out or the person becomes unconscious.

 For Someone in a Wheelchair:

1. Lock the wheels of the wheelchair.

2. Kneel or crouch behind the person.

3. Wrap both arms around the bulk of the wheelchair and the abdomen.

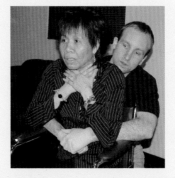

4. Make a fist with one hand and place the thumb side of the fist just above the belly button.

5. Grasp your fist with your other hand.

6. Pull sharply in and up.

7. Continue until the object comes out or the person becomes unconscious.

Choking Alone

1. Dial EMS/9-1-1 and leave the phone off the hook. This will tell the dispatcher to send help.

2. If there may be people nearby, move to a place where you can get yourself noticed.

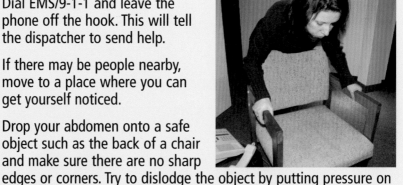

3. Drop your abdomen onto a safe object such as the back of a chair and make sure there are no sharp edges or corners. Try to dislodge the object by putting pressure on the same area you would use for abdominal thrusts.

Baby

Check:

- Check the scene for danger.

- If it is safe to do so, check the baby.

Call:

- Shout for help.

Care:

1. If a baby is coughing or gagging the choking is mild. Do not interfere.

2. If the baby is making high-pitched noises, wheezing, can no longer make a sound or becomes too weak to cough:

  - Send someone to call EMS/9-1-1.

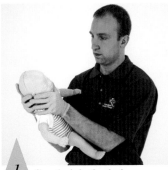

1 Sandwich the baby between your forearms, supporting the head.

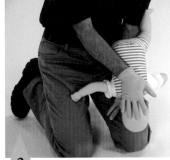

2 Turn the baby face down with the head lower than the body.

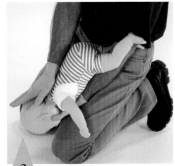

3 Lower your forearm onto your thigh. With the heel of your hand, deliver five back blows between the shoulder blades.

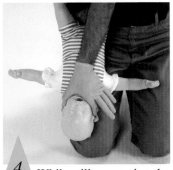

4 While still supporting the head, turn the baby face up, with your arm supported on your thigh.

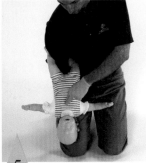

5 Place two fingers on the middle of the chest just below the nipple line and "push hard, push fast" 1/3 to 1/2 the depth of the chest five times.

6 Repeat the back blows and chest thrusts until the object is coughed up; the baby starts to cry, breathe, or cough; or the baby becomes unconscious.

If the object comes out or the baby starts to cry, breathe, or cough:

Secondary Survey:

Perform a secondary survey and treat any non-life-threatening injuries.

Continual Care:

Provide continual care.

If the baby becomes unconscious:

Follow the steps for unconscious choking later in this chapter.

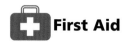 **First Aid**

Unconscious Choking

Adult or Child

Check:

- Check the scene for danger.
- If it is safe to do so, check the person.

NOTE:

"Push hard, push fast."
Compression depths:
Adult – 4 to 5 cm (1.5 to 2 in)
Child or baby – 1/3 to 1/2
the depth of the chest

Call:

- If the person does not respond, have someone call EMS/9-1-1 and get an AED (automated external defibrillator) if one is available. If you are alone with an adult, call EMS/9-1-1 yourself, then return to care for the person. If you are alone with a child, do 5 cycles (two minutes) of CPR first, then go call EMS/9-1-1 and return to care for the child.

Care:

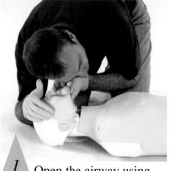

1 Open the airway using the head-tilt/chin-lift and check for normal breathing for 5 to 10 seconds:

- Look, listen, and feel.

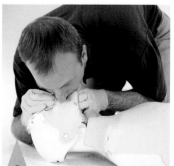

2 If you do not hear normal breathing, give two rescue breaths:

- Pinch the nose.
- Take a normal breath.
- Cover the person's mouth with your mouth.
- Give two breaths; each breath should last one second, with enough volume to make the chest rise.

3 If the person's chest does not rise after the first breath, perform the head-tilt/chin-lift again. Try tilting the head further back and attempt to give a breath.

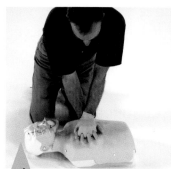

4 If your breath still does not go in, start CPR:

- Place the heel of one hand in the middle of the person's chest. Place the other hand on top.
- Do 30 compressions. "Push hard, push fast."
- Allow the chest to recoil.

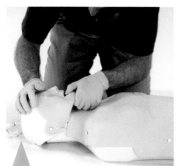

5a After each cycle of compressions, look in the mouth.

- Grasp both the tongue and lower jaw and lift.
- If you do not see an object, try to give a breath, if breath does not go in, go to Step 4.
- If you see an object, remove it and go to Step 6.

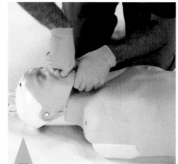

5b • Slide your finger down the inside of the cheek to the base of the tongue and try to sweep the object out.

NOTE:

If your breath does not go in, go back to compressions.

NOTE:

If there is any change in the person's condition during CPR, stop and check the person's ABCs.

6 Give a breath. If your first breath goes in, give a second breath.

7 When both breaths go in, and there is no obvious response to your two breaths, start the CPR sequence of 30 compressions and 2 breaths.

Baby

Check:

- Check the scene for danger.
- If it is safe to do so, check the baby.

Call:

- If the baby does not respond, have someone call EMS/9-1-1. If you are alone with a baby, do 5 cycles (two minutes) of CPR first, then take the baby with you (as long as you don't suspect a head or spine injury) to call EMS/9-1-1.

Care:

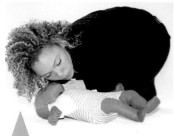

1 Open the airway using the head-tilt/chin-lift and check for normal breathing for 5 to 10 seconds:

- Look, listen, and feel.

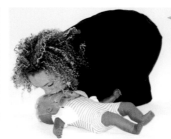

2 If you do not hear normal breathing, give two gentle breaths:

- Take a normal breath.
- Seal your lips tightly over the baby's mouth and nose.
- Give two breaths; each breath should last one second, with just enough volume to make the chest rise.

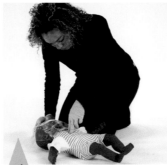

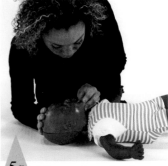

3 If the baby's chest does not rise after the first breath, perform the head-tilt/chin-lift again and attempt to give a breath.

4 If your breath still does not go in, start CPR:

- Place two fingers on the middle of the chest, just below the nipple line.
- Do 30 compressions. "Push hard, push fast."
- Allow the chest to recoil.

5a After each cycle of compressions, look in the mouth.

- Grasp both the tongue and lower jaw and lift.
- If you do not see an object, try to give a breath, if breath does not go in, go to Step 4.
- If you can see an object, remove it and go to Step 6.

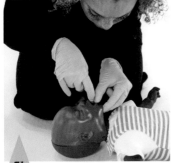

5b Slide your finger down the inside of the cheek to the base of the tongue and try to sweep the object out.

6 Give a breath. If your first breath goes in, give a second breath.

7 When both breaths go in and if there is no obvious response to your two breaths, start the CPR sequence of 30 compressions and 2 breaths.

NOTE:
If there is any change in the baby's condition during CPR, stop and check the baby's ABCs.

NOTE:
If your breath does not go in, go back to compressions.

Breathing and Circulation Emergencies

Breathing and Circulation Emergencies

After a very fast-paced shift on the soccer field, a teenaged player cannot catch her breath. The condition gets worse very quickly, and she loses consciousness and collapses at the side of the field.

BREATHING EMERGENCIES

A person having difficulty breathing is in ***respiratory distress***. A person who can't breathe at all is in ***respiratory arrest***. Both respiratory distress and respiratory arrest are ***breathing emergencies***. Brain cells begin to die in four to six minutes without oxygen (Figure 6.1).

0 minute: Breathing stops. Heart will soon stop beating. Clinical death.

4–6 minutes: Brain damage possible.

6–10 minutes: Brain damage likely.

10+ minutes: Irreversible brain damage certain. Biological death.

Figure 6.1 Four to six minutes without oxygen generally causes brain damage.

COMMON CAUSES OF RESPIRATORY DISTRESS

- Hyperventilation
- Asthma
- Allergic reaction or anaphylaxis
- Chest injury

HYPERVENTILATION

Hyperventilation occurs when breathing is faster than normal. This upsets the body's balance of oxygen and carbon dioxide.

▶ Causes of Hyperventilation

- Emotion, such as excitement, fear, or anxiety
- Some medical conditions
- Injury

Prevention of Hyperventilation

If you tend to hyperventilate due to anxiety, panic, or stress, practise breathing exercises or relaxation techniques.

If you hyperventilate due to an underlying medical condition, a doctor will help you understand and treat your condition.

 Signs and Symptoms of Hyperventilation

- Rapid, shallow breathing
- A feeling of suffocating or not getting enough air
- Fear, anxiety, or confusion
- Dizziness and numbness or tingling of fingers and toes

 First Aid for Hyperventilation

Check:

- Check the scene for danger.
- If it is safe to do so, check the person.

Call:

- Have someone call EMS/9-1-1 if there are signs and symptoms of an injury or an underlying illness or condition, the hyperventilation does not stop after a few minutes, or the person becomes unconscious. If you are alone, call EMS/9-1-1 yourself, then return to care for the person.

Care:

1 Make sure ABCs are present.

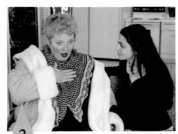

2 Tell the person to relax and breathe slowly. You can often stop hyperventilation by reassuring the person.

Secondary Survey:

Perform a secondary survey and treat any non-life-threatening injuries.

Continual Care:

Provide continual care until EMS personnel arrive.

ASTHMA

During an asthma attack, the air passages become narrower and breathing is difficult. Asthma is more common in children. It is usually controlled with medication.

 Preventing Asthma Attacks

If you have asthma:

- Know what causes an asthma attack (such as strenuous exercise, cold weather, stress, or allergens) and avoid it if possible.

- Always have your medication nearby in case of an attack.

If your child has asthma:

- Make sure that anyone who supervises your child knows about the asthma and how to help give medication if necessary.

 Signs and Symptoms of Asthma

During an asthma attack, a person may:

- Wheeze when exhaling

- Be gasping for air or seem unable to catch his breath

- Be upset

- Feel his chest tightening or feel tingling in the hands and feet

 First Aid for Asthma

Check:

- Check the scene for danger.

- If it is safe to do so, check the person.

Call:

- Have someone call EMS/9-1-1 if the person is struggling to breathe or if the person is not responding to his medication. If you are alone, call EMS/9-1-1 yourself, then return to care for the person.

Care:

1. Calm the person down to help slow down his breathing.

2. Help the person take any prescribed medication for his condition.

Secondary Survey:

Perform a secondary survey and treat any non-life-threatening injuries:

1. Move the person away from the environment if this is what caused the attack.

2. Help the person get into a comfortable position.

Continual Care:

Provide continual care.

▶ How to Help Someone Use an Inhaler (Puffer) With a Spacer[1]

1. Make sure that you have the inhaler that has been pre-scribed to that particular person (Figure 6.2).

2. Shake the inhaler three or four times.

3. Remove the cap from the inhaler. If the person uses a spacer and it has a cap, remove it.

4. If the person uses a spacer, put the inhaler into the spacer.

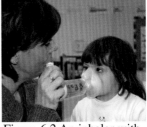

Figure 6.2 An inhaler with spacer.

5. Have the person breathe out, away from the inhaler and spacer.

6. Bring the spacer or inhaler to the person's mouth, put the mouthpiece between her teeth, and tell the person to close her lips around it.

NOTE:

Some spacers come in the form of a mask.

7. Tell the person to press the top of the inhaler once. If the person can't do it, you may do it instead.

8. Tell the person to take one slow, full breath, hold it for about 10 seconds, and then breathe out.

[1]Adapted from www.lung.ca

ALLERGIC REACTIONS

Allergic reactions are sensitivities to specific substances that can be absorbed through the skin, inhaled into the lungs, swallowed, or injected.

 Preventing Allergic Reactions

- If you have an allergy to food, read ingredient labels carefully, and when eating out, ask questions about what is in the food.

- Avoid triggers such as foods and medications that have caused any type of allergic reaction in the past.

- If you have a child who is allergic to certain foods, introduce one new food at a time so you can recognize an allergic reaction.

 Signs and Symptoms of Allergic Reactions

- Previous allergic episodes

- Rash, itching, or hives (raised, itchy areas of skin) (Figure 6.3)

- A feeling of tightness in the chest and throat

- Swelling of the lips, face, ears, neck, and/or tongue

- Abnormal breathing sounds, such as wheezing or high-pitched noises

- Weakness, dizziness, or confusion

- Nausea or vomiting

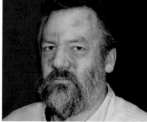

Figure 6.3 Rash, itching, or hives are a sign of an allergic reaction.

 First Aid for Allergic Reactions

Check:

- Check the scene for danger.

- If it is safe to do so, check the person.

Call:

- Have someone call EMS/9-1-1 if the reaction is severe, if the person is struggling to breathe, or if the person loses consciousness. If you are alone, call EMS/9-1-1 yourself, then return to care for the person.

Care:

- Make sure ABCs are present.

Secondary Survey:

Perform a secondary survey and treat any non-life-threatening injuries:

1. Calm and reassure the person having the reaction as anxiety can worsen symptoms.

2. Try to identify the allergen and have the person avoid further contact with it.

3. If the person develops an itchy rash, apply calamine lotion and cool compresses.

4. Watch the person for signs of increasing distress.

Continual Care:

Provide continual care. Seek medical attention. For a mild reaction, a doctor may recommend over-the-counter medications (such as antihistamines).

ANAPHYLAXIS

Anaphylaxis is a severe allergic reaction. The air passages may swell, making breathing difficult. In some cases the person may go into respiratory arrest. Anaphylaxis may be caused by insect stings, food, medications, or other allergens.

 Preventing Anaphylaxis

- Be careful to avoid the substances, foods, or insects that cause a reaction.

- If you know that you have a severe allergy (anaphylaxis), wear a MedicAlert® medical identification product and carry your medication with you.

- Parents of a child with severe allergies must be especially vigilant and tell anyone looking after their child of the allergies and the possible reactions.

Signs and Symptoms of Anaphylaxis

The signs and symptoms of anaphylaxis are similar to the signs and symptoms of an allergic reaction, but they are more pronounced:

- Swelling of the lips, ears, and/or hands
- Generalized redness of the skin—this is often a raised, itchy, blotchy rash or hives
- Weakness or dizziness
- Nausea or vomiting
- Breathing difficulty, coughing, and wheezing. Tongue and throat swelling may block the airway

First Aid for Anaphylaxis

Check:

1. Check the scene for danger.
2. If it is safe to do so, check the person.

Call:

- Have someone call EMS/9-1-1. If you are alone, call EMS/9-1-1 yourself, then return to care for the person.

Care:

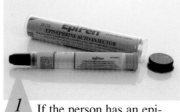

1 If the person has an epinephrine auto-injector, help her use it.

Secondary Survey:

Perform a secondary survey and treat any non-life-threatening injuries:

1. Calm the person down to help slow down her breathing.
2. Help the person get into a comfortable position.

Continual Care:

Provide continual care until EMS personnel arrive.

▶ **How to Use an Epinephrine Auto-Injector**

△ *1* Make sure that you check the five rights of medication (see the Five Rights of Medication on page 63).

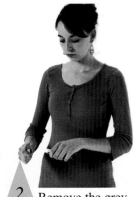

△ *2* Remove the grey safety cap.

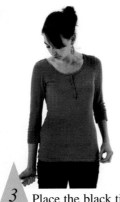

△ *3* Place the black tip against the person's outer thigh and push the epinephrine auto-injector firmly against the thigh with a quick motion. You should hear a click. Hold for 10 seconds.

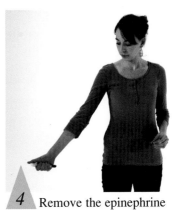

△ *4* Remove the epinephrine auto-injector.

Make sure the used epinephrine auto-injector goes with the person to the hospital.

RESPIRATORY ARREST

A person who stops breathing is in ***respiratory arrest***. Without prompt first aid, respiratory distress can lead to respiratory arrest.

▶ **Causes of Respiratory Arrest**

- Electrocution
- Drowning
- Drugs and alcohol
- Injury to the head, chest, or lungs
- Suffocation
- Strangulation
- Airway obstructions
- A severe allergic reaction to food or an insect sting
- Respiratory conditions (such as emphysema or asthma)
- Poisoning, such as inhaling or swallowing something toxic

▶ **Signs and Symptoms of Respiratory Arrest**

- Unconsciousness

- Bluish-coloured lips and a face that is paler than normal

- Lack of movement in the chest and abdomen, except for the occasional attempt to breathe

- Lack of breathing sounds, except for the occasional gasp or gurgle

First aid for respiratory arrest is found in Chapter 7 (or Chapter 8 if you're a healthcare provider).

CIRCULATION EMERGENCIES

During coffee break at the warehouse where you work, one of the forklift drivers complains about pain in his chest. You notice that he is looking pale and is sweating.

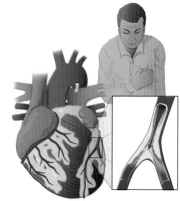

HEART ATTACK

A *heart attack* happens when the heart can't get enough oxygen because of a blockage in one of the arteries feeding the heart muscle (Figure 6.4). A heart attack is caused by *cardiovascular disease*. Cardiovascular disease is any disease that affects the heart or the blood vessels.

Figure 6.4 A heart attack.

▶ **Risk Factors for Developing Cardiovascular Disease**

Controllable factors:

- Smoking

- Poor diet (especially a diet that is high in cholesterol)

- High blood pressure

- Obesity

CPR Adult or Child

Check the scene

Call for help

 Care

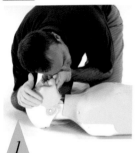 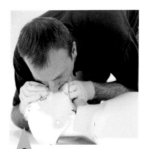 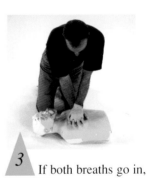

1 Open the airway and check for normal breathing for 5 to 10 seconds.

2 If you do not hear normal breathing, give two rescue breaths.

3 If both breaths go in, start CPR:

- Do 30 compressions : 2 breaths. "Push hard, push fast."

- Continue until help arrives.

Canadian Red Cross   1-877-356-3226 | www.redcross.ca

Over for AED

CPR Adult or Child

AED

When the AED Arrives:

1. Open and turn on the AED.

2. Remove any clothing or objects that interfere with pad placement.

3. Ensure that the chest is dry and free of hair.

4. Follow the diagrams on the pad for placement.

5. Follow the automated prompts of the AED.

6. When the AED prompts you to give a shock, stand clear and say, "I'm clear, you're clear, everybody's clear."

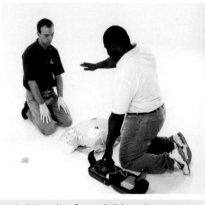

A child is between the ages of one and eight. For a child use child pads. If no child pads are available, use adult pads. Follow the directions on the pads for placement.

If there is less than 2.5 cm (1 in) between pads when on the chest, place one on the front of the chest and one on the back.

For other considerations refer to the **Red Cross** *First Aid & CPR Manual.*

CPR for Baby

Check the scene

Call for help

 Care

NOTE:

If you are alone do 5 cycles of CPR, then take the baby with you to call EMS/9-1-1.

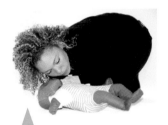

1 Open the airway and check for normal breathing for 5 to 10 seconds.

NOTE:

Do not tilt the head back too far.

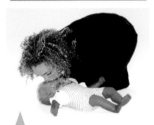

2 If you do not hear normal breathing, give two gentle breaths.

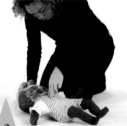

3 If both breaths go in, start CPR:
- Place two fingers on the middle of the chest, just below the nipple line.
- Do 30 compressions : 2 breaths. "Push hard, push fast."
- Continue until help arrives.

 Canadian Red Cross   1-877-356-3226 | www.redcross.ca

Why the Heart Stops

In babies, cardiac arrest is most often due to respiratory arrest.

Causes

- Strangulation/suffocation
- Poisoning
- Airway obstruction
- Drowning
- Electrocution

Prevention

- Use pacifier clips, not cords
- Supervise babies nursing on a bottle
- Keep choking hazards away from babies
- Pay constant attention to babies when they are in or near water
- Keep babies away from pillows
- Use electrical wall protection plugs

 Canadian Red Cross   1-877-356-3226 | www.redcross.ca

Check, Call, Care

Local Emergency Number: _____

Poison Control Centre: _____

Doctor's Number: _____

Dentist's Number: _____

Our Contact Information
Address: _____
Nearest Main Intersection: _____
Phone: _____
Neighbour's Name: _____
Neighbour's Phone: _____

Check, Call, Care

SECONDARY SURVEY

If the person's ABCs are present, you need to find out what else may be wrong. To do this, you should do a secondary survey of the person to look for injuries that are not life-threatening at this point in time.

 Ask Questions

Get more information by asking the SAMPLE questions:

S = Signs and symptoms

A = Allergies

M = Medications

P = Past medical history

L = Last meal

E = Events leading up to the emergency

 Check Vital Signs

Level of consciousness Is the person awake or sleepy? Does the person seem confused? Is the person responsive?

Breathing Listen for sounds. Is the breathing fast or slow, shallow or deep? Is breathing painful for the person?

Skin Is it dry or wet? Is it an unusual colour or temperature?

Conscious Choking Adult or Child

Check the scene

- If the person is coughing or gagging, the choking is mild, do not interfere

Call for help

- If the person is making a high-pitched noise, wheezing, can no longer make a sound or becomes too weak to cough:

  Send someone to call for help

 Care

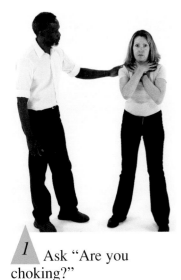

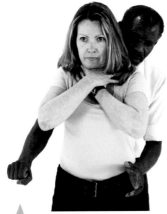

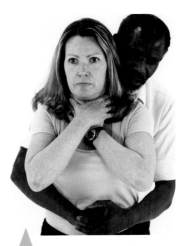

1 Ask "Are you choking?"

2 Stand (or kneel for a small child) behind the person and wrap both arms around the abdomen.

3 Make a fist and place it just above the belly button.

- Place your other hand over the fist.
- Pull sharply in and up.

Continue until:

- Object comes out or
- Person becomes unconscious

Follow the steps for unconscious choking

Canadian Red Cross   1-877-356-3226 | www.redcross.ca

Unconscious Choking Adult or Child

Check the scene

Call for help

• Have someone call EMS/9-1-1.

If you are alone: Adult – call EMS/9-1-1 yourself and then return to care for the person.

Child – do 5 cycles of CPR first, then go call EMS/9-1-1 and return to care for the child.

 Care

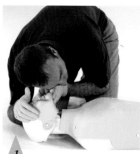

1 Open airway using the head-tilt/chin-lift. Check for normal breathing for 5 to 10 seconds.

• Look, listen, and feel.

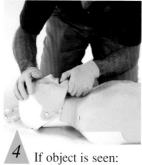

4 If object is seen:

• Lift the jaw.

• Slide your finger down inside of the cheek to the base of the tongue to sweep object out.

• Give a breath. If it goes in, give a second breath. When breaths go in, and there is no obvious response, start CPR sequence of 30 compressions : 2 breaths.

2 If no normal breathing, give rescue breaths:

• Pinch the nose.

• Cover the person's mouth with your mouth.

• Give two breaths. Each lasting one second, with enough volume to make the chest rise.

• If chest does not rise after the first breath try retilting the head.

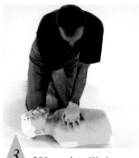

3 If breath still does not go in, start CPR:

• Do 30 compressions.

• "Push hard, push fast."

• Adult–compress 4 to 5 cm (1.5-2 in)

• Child–compress 1/3 to 1/2 the chest depth

After each cycle of compressions, look in the mouth. If no object is seen, try to give a breath. If breath does not go in, go back to CPR.

Canadian Red Cross   1-877-356-3226 | www.redcross.ca

Conscious Choking Baby

Check the scene

- If a baby is coughing or gagging, the choking is mild, do not interfere.

Call for help

- If the baby is making high-pitched noises, wheezing, no longer making a sound or becomes too weak to cough:

Send someone to call for help.

 Care

1 Sandwich the baby between your forearms, supporting the head.

2 Turn the baby face down with the head lower than the body

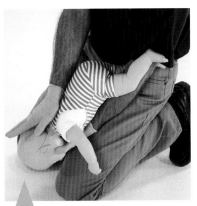

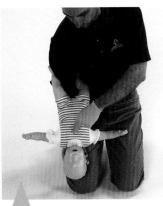

3 Lower your forearm onto your thigh. With the heel of your hand, deliver five back blows between the shoulder blades.

4 Place two fingers on the middle of the chest just below the nipple line and "push hard, push fast", 5 times.

- Repeat the back blows and chest thrusts until the object is coughed up; the baby starts to cry, breathe, or cough; or the baby becomes unconscious.

If the baby becomes unconscious, follow the steps for unconscious choking on the back.

Canadian Red Cross   1-877-356-3226 | www.redcross.ca

Unconscious Choking Baby

Check the scene

Call for help

 Care

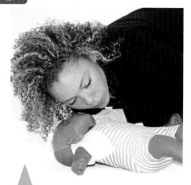

1 Open the airway and check for normal breathing for 5 to 10 seconds.

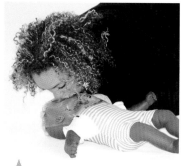

2 If you do not hear normal breathing, give two gentle breaths.

3 If the baby's chest does not rise after the first breath, perform the head-tilt/chin-lift again, and attempt to give a breath.

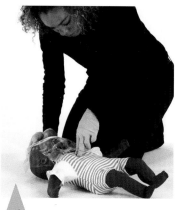

4 If your breath still does not go in, start CPR:
- Do 30 compressions. "Push hard, push fast." Allow the chest to recoil.

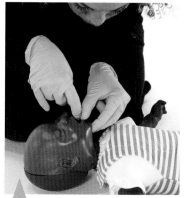

5 After each cycle of compressions, look in the mouth.
- Grasp both the tongue and lower jaw and lift.
- If you do not see an object, try to give a breath, if breath does not go in, go to Step 4.
- If you see an object, remove it and go to Step 6.

6 Give a breath. If your first breath goes in, give a second breath.

7 If there is no obvious response to your two breaths, start CPR.

Canadian Red Cross   1-877-356-3226 | www.redcross.ca

- Stress
- Lack of regular exercise

Other factors:

- Gender
- Heredity
- Age

 Preventing Heart Attacks

Although a heart attack may seem to strike suddenly, cardiovascular disease develops over a long period of time. In fact, it can begin as early as the teenage years.

To prevent cardiovascular disease and heart attacks, you should follow the guidelines for a healthy lifestyle described below.

 Nutrition

A healthy lifestyle starts with a healthy, balanced diet. Each day you should have something from the four basic food groups: grain products, vegetables and fruits, milk products, and meat and alternatives. Check Canada's Food Guide to find out how much you should be eating from each food group.

Keep these points in mind as well:

- Fluids are important. Drink plenty of water each day. Eight 8 oz glasses (236 mL) each day are recommended.

- Fibre is important. Good sources include whole-grain breads and cereals, fruits, and leafy vegetables.

- Avoid foods that are high in salt, fat, and cholesterol (such as burgers, fries, etc.).

NOTE:
It is important to have some salt in your diet.

To improve your eating habits:

- Know the food you buy. Read the labels!

- Try choosing "light" dairy products or a low-fat substitute for high-fat dairy products.

- Use non-hydrogenated oils and fats for cooking.

Weight Control

Having too much body fat can lead to heart disease, high blood pressure, diabetes, and gallbladder disease.

Losing weight, especially fat, is not easy. Your weight depends on the balance between how much you eat and how many calories you use through the day. However, other factors can also affect your weight, including thyroid problems, hormones, and when you eat.

To lose body fat:

• Get your body fat percentage checked by a certified trainer or doctor.

• Eat fewer calories than you use, but try to lose body fat only gradually.

• Exercise regularly. Exercise is a key part of controlling your body fat.

▶ **Exercise**

Exercise is good for the heart, lungs, blood vessels, and muscles. Even if you don't have a lot of time for exercise, try to increase your cardiovascular fitness. This helps you:

• Cope with everyday stress

• Improve your self-esteem

• Control your body fat

• Sleep better

• Fight infections

Try to exercise at least three times a week for 20 to 30 minutes at your target heart rate. This rate is 65 to 80 percent of your maximum heart rate, which goes down as you get older. Talk to your doctor or fitness trainer to plan a proper training program.

Turn your daily activities into exercise. Look for ways to make exercise fun so that it is easier to make it a regular habit. If you have not been active, or if you have health problems, see your doctor before you start an exercise program.

▶ **Stress Control**

Stress is a normal part of life. If you learn how to cope with it well, you can help prevent illness and stay healthy. To reduce stress:

• Develop rewarding hobbies.

• Exercise regularly.

• Avoid coffee, tea, chocolate, soft drinks, or pain relievers that contain caffeine, which all reduce your ability to handle stress.

• Set goals that you can reach. Unrealistic goals will only add to your stress.

- Practise relaxation exercises. Sit or lie quietly in a comfortable position with your eyes closed. Breathe in deeply through your nose and out through your mouth. Focus on your breathing for 10 minutes.

▶ Breaking Unhealthy Habits: Smoking

In the past few decades the dangers of smoking have become well known. Smoking is banned or restricted in many work sites and public places.

Smoking tobacco is the most preventable cause of heart disease. Smoking also causes most cases of lung cancer, and it can lead to other forms of respiratory distress. Fortunately, the risk of respiratory and cardiovascular problems starts to drop as soon as you stop smoking.

Smokeless tobacco is also dangerous. Chewing tobacco and snuff cause cancer of the mouth, tongue, and nasal passages.

There are many programs available to help smokers break the habit. Contact your local public health unit for more information.

▶ Signs and Symptoms of a Heart Attack

- Squeezing chest pain

- Problems breathing

- Abdominal or back pain (most commonly in women)

- Cold, sweaty skin

- Skin that is bluish or paler than normal

- Nausea and vomiting

- Denial

During a heart attack many women, elderly people, and diabetics tend to experience "soft signs," including:

- Mild, unfocussed chest discomfort that:
    - ▶ Comes and goes
    - ▶ Doesn't feel like pain
    - ▶ Starts mild and gets continually stronger
    - ▶ Gets better with rest
    - ▶ Gets worse with activity

- Tiredness

- Gastric discomfort

- Flu-like symptoms

NOTE:

Some men have these signs as well.

ANGINA

Angina is chest pain or pressure that comes and goes.

▶ Causes of Angina

- Cardiovascular disease

- Anemia

- Certain heart disorders

▶ Signs and Symptoms of Angina

The signs and symptoms of angina are similar to the signs and symptoms of a heart attack, but:

- The pain usually lasts less than 10 minutes.

- The pain usually goes away if the person rests.

First Aid for Heart Attack and Angina

Check:

- Check the scene for danger.

- If it is safe to do so, check the person.

Call:

- If the signs and symptoms don't go away with rest and/or nitroglycerin, have someone call EMS/9-1-1. If you are alone, call EMS/9-1-1 yourself, then return to care for the person.

Care:

1. Have the person rest comfortably.

2. Ask the person if he or she has taken any drugs for erectile dysfunction (such as Viagra®, Levitra®, or Cialis®). If he or she has, do not allow him or her to take nitroglycerin.

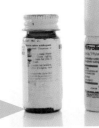

3. Help the person take nitroglycerin (if he or she has it) and ASA.

- Nitroglycerin can come as a spray or pill. Nitroglycerin is placed or sprayed under the tongue.

If someone is unconscious, never put anything in his or her mouth.

4. The nitroglycerin dose may be repeated every five minutes until the pain is relieved or until a maximum of three doses has been administered.

   - If the person doesn't carry nitroglycerin, or if the first dose of nitroglycerin doesn't make the pain go away, suggest that the person chew two chewable ASA tablets (80 mg each) or one regular-strength adult ASA tablet (325 mg).

> **NOTE:**
>
> *ASA won't make the pain go away, but it helps stop clotting in the arteries, thus reducing damage to the heart. Do not repeat the dosage. Medications such as acetaminophen (e.g., Tylenol®) or ibuprofen (e.g., Advil®) **do not** have the same effect as ASA in reducing damage due to heart attacks. Do not substitute!*

Secondary Survey:

Perform a secondary survey and treat any non-life-threatening injuries.

Continual Care:

Provide continual care until EMS personnel arrive.

Before offering ASA, ask if the person has an allergy to it or has asthma. If the answer to either question is yes, do not give ASA.

Five Rights of Medication

1. **Right person:** Make sure the person getting the medication is the one whose name is on the label of the medicine container.

2. **Right medication:** Read the label when you are getting the medication.

3. **Right amount:** Use an accurately marked measuring container (if applicable).

4. **Right time:** Give the medication at the right time.

5. **Right method:** Read the directions carefully.

CARDIAC ARREST

Cardiac arrest occurs when the heart stops beating.

Causes of Cardiac Arrest

Cardiovascular disease is the most common cause of cardiac arrest. Other common causes include:

- Drowning
- Suffocation
- Certain drugs
- Other heart diseases or abnormalities
- Severe blood loss
- Electrocution
- Severe chest injuries

▶ Signs and Symptoms of Cardiac Arrest

- Unconsciousness
- No signs of normal breathing

First Aid: CPR/AED for Cardiac Arrest

Because the brain and other vital organs can live for only a few minutes after the heart stops beating, someone in cardiac arrest needs CPR, defibrillation, and advanced emergency medical care as soon as possible.

CPR combines rescue breaths and chest compressions to keep oxygen-rich blood circulating throughout the body. CPR will keep a minimal amount of blood moving to the vital organs until an AED is available and EMS personnel arrive.

NOTE:

An AED should not be used on a baby.

An AED is a machine that analyzes the heart's electrical rhythm and, if necessary, tells the user to deliver a shock to the person in cardiac arrest. This is called **defibrillation.** The shock helps the heart re-establish an effective rhythm.

Studies show that if you can defibrillate someone quickly, the chance of survival increases greatly. For each minute that someone has to wait for defibrillation, the chance of survival drops about 7 to 10 percent.[1]

Public Access Defibrillation (PAD) is a movement to make AEDs readily available in many public areas, such as arenas or shopping centres. The advantage of AEDs is that it doesn't take intensive training to use them. With a little training and with voice prompts from the machine, users can successfully defibrillate someone in cardiac arrest. Contact your local city or municipality to find out if there is a PAD program in your area.

[1]The American Heart Association in collaboration with the International Liaison Committee on Resuscitation. "Guidelines 2000 for Cardiopulmonary Resuscitation and Emergency Cardiovascular Care: International Consensus on Science, Part 4: the Automated External Defibrillator: Key Link in the Chain of Survival." Circulation, 2000; 102 (Suppl I):I-60–76.

STROKE

A **stroke** happens when the blood flow to the brain gets interrupted (Figure 6.5).

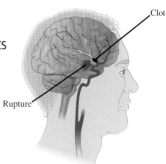

Causes of a Stroke

- A clot in an artery in the brain

- An artery that bursts in the brain

- A tumour

Figure 6.5 A stroke can be caused by a clot or a rupture.

Preventing Stroke

The risk factors for stroke are similar to those for heart disease. You can help prevent stroke with the same lifestyle changes discussed in the earlier section on preventing cardiovascular disease.

Signs and Symptoms of a Stroke

Remember FAST:

FACE — facial numbness or weakness, especially on one side (Figure 6.6)

ARM — arm numbness or weakness, especially on one side

SPEECH — slurred speech or difficulty speaking or under standing

TIME — time is important; call EMS/9-1-1 immediately

NOTE:

Other signs and symptoms include:
- *a sudden, severe headache*
- *dizziness or confusion*
- *unconsciousness or temporary loss of consciousness*
- *sudden loss of bladder control*

First Aid for a Stroke

Check:

- Check the scene for danger.

- If it is safe to do so, check the person.

Call:

- Have someone call EMS/9-1-1. If you are alone, call EMS/9-1-1 yourself, then return to care for the person.

Care:

1. Make sure ABCs are present.

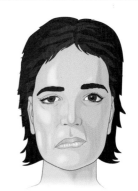

Figure 6.6 Facial numbness or weakness.

Secondary Survey:

Perform a secondary survey and treat any non-life-threatening injuries.

Continual Care:

Have the person rest. Place the person in the recovery position with the affected side up, if possible. Monitor the ABCs. Reassure the person until EMS personnel arrive because this can be an extremely frightening experience.

TRANSIENT ISCHEMIC ATTACK (TIA)

A *transient ischemic attack* (TIA) is like a "mini-stroke," caused by a temporary drop in blood flow to part of the brain.

NOTE:

You can prevent TIAs in the same way you can prevent strokes.

 Causes of a TIA

- A clot in an artery in the brain
- An artery that bursts in the brain
- A tumour

 Signs and Symptoms of a TIA

The signs and symptoms of a TIA are the same as the signs and symptoms of a stroke, but they disappear within a few minutes or hours.

NOTE:

Angina and TIAs are very similar. Both are a temporary drop in the flow of oxygen-rich blood to a vital organ. Angina is a drop in blood flow to the heart, whereas a TIA is a drop in blood flow to the brain.

 First Aid for a TIA

Follow the same steps as "First Aid for a Stroke."

DEADLY BLEEDING

Deadly bleeding leads to large amounts of blood loss, either outside or within the body.

▶ Preventing Deadly Bleeding

- Be familiar with your surroundings.
- Keep all sharp objects, such as knives, in a safe place.
- Be aware of any machinery in the workplace.
- Wear appropriate safety equipment at work.
- Be familiar with your equipment.
- Get proper training on machinery in the workplace.
- Stay alert.

▶ Signs and Symptoms of External Deadly Bleeding

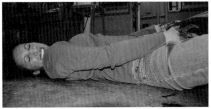

- Large amounts of bleeding (Figure 6.7)
- Signs of shock

Figure 6.7 Deadly bleeding.

First Aid for External Deadly Bleeding

Check:

- Check the scene for danger.
- If it is safe to do so, check the person.

Call:

- Have someone call EMS/9-1-1. If you are alone, call EMS/9-1-1 yourself, then return to care for the person.

REMEMBER:
Wear personal protective equipment.

Care:

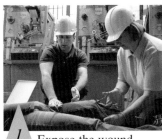

1 Expose the wound.

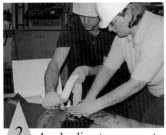

2 Apply direct pressure to the bleeding.

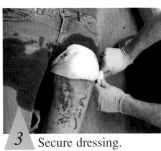

3 Secure dressing.

Secondary Survey:

Perform a secondary survey and treat any non-life-threatening injuries.

Continual Care:

Provide continual care until EMS personnel arrive.

 Signs and Symptoms of Internal Deadly Bleeding

- Bruising in the injured area (Figure 6.8)

- Soft tissues (such as the abdomen) that are tender, swollen, or hard

- Shock

- Blood in saliva or vomit

- Pain

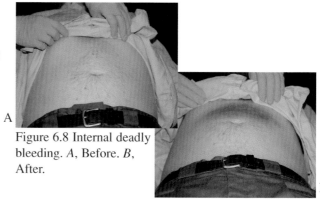

A

Figure 6.8 Internal deadly bleeding. *A*, Before. *B*, After.

NOTE:

You should suspect internal bleeding in any injury that involved a forceful blow to the body.

Internal bleeding is more difficult to recognize than external bleeding because the signs and symptoms are less obvious and they may take longer to appear.

NOTE:

Remember your gloves and other barrier devices.

 First Aid for Internal Deadly Bleeding

Check:

- Check the scene for danger.

- If it is safe to do so, check the person.

Call:

- Have someone call EMS/9-1-1. If you are alone, call EMS/9-1-1 yourself, then return to care for the person.

Care:

- Help the person rest in the most comfortable position.

Secondary Survey:

Perform a secondary survey and treat any non-life-threatening injuries.

Continual Care:

Provide continual care until EMS personnel arrive.

First Aid for Respiratory and Cardiac Arrest

First Aid for Respiratory and Cardiac Arrest

ROLLING A PERSON

If someone is face down and you cannot check if she is breathing in that position, you will need to roll the person over:

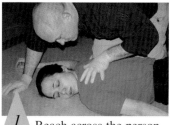

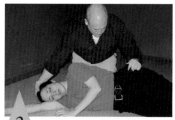

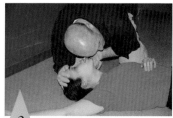

 1 Reach across the person and grab any clothing close to the waist that is strong enough to pull on.

2 Try to support the head and neck while rolling the person to prevent the head from hitting the floor. Roll the person towards you.

3 Once you have the person on her back, open the airway and check breathing.

First Aid for Respiratory and Cardiac Arrest

Adult or Child

Check:

• Check the scene for danger.

• If it is safe to do so, check the person.

Call:

• If the person does not respond, have someone call EMS/9-1-1 and get an AED if one is available. If you are alone with an adult, call EMS/9-1-1 yourself, then return to care for the person. If you are alone with a child, do 5 cycles (two minutes) of CPR first, then call EMS/9-1-1 and return to care for the child.

Care:

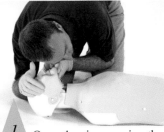

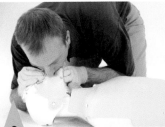

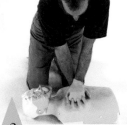

1 Open the airway using the head-tilt/chin-lift and check for normal breathing for 5 to 10 seconds:

• Look, listen, and feel.

2 If you do not hear normal breathing, give two rescue breaths:

• Pinch the nose.

• Take a normal breath.

• Cover the person's mouth with your mouth.

• Give two breaths. Each breath should last one second, with enough volume to make the chest rise.

3 If both breaths go in, start CPR:

• Place the heel of one hand in the middle of the person's chest. Place the other hand on top.

• Do 30 compressions. "Push hard, push fast."

• Allow the chest to recoil.

• Repeat cycle of compressions and breaths.

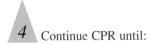

4 Continue CPR until:

• An AED arrives.

• More advanced care takes over.

• The scene becomes unsafe.

• You become physically unable to continue.

> **NOTE:**
>
> *"Push hard, push fast."*
> *Compression depths:*
> *Adult – 4 to 5 cm (1.5 to 2 in)*
> *Child or baby – 1/3 to 1/2*
> *the depth of the chest*

When the AED Arrives:

1. Open and turn on the AED.

2. Remove any clothing or objects (including jewellery or medical patches) from the person that may come in contact with the pads.

3. Ensure that the chest is dry and free of hair so the pads can stick.

4. Follow the diagrams on the pads to place them on the person. Use the appropriate pad based on the person — adult or child.

5. Follow the automated prompts of the AED.

6. When the AED prompts you to give a shock (Figure 7.1), stand clear and say, "I'm clear, you're clear, everybody's clear."

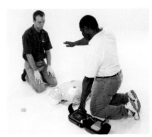

Figure 7.1 Stand clear.

A child is between the ages of one and eight. If no child pads are available, use adult pads. Follow the directions for pad placement.

If there is less than 2.5 cm (1 in) between the pads when on the chest, place one on the front of the chest (anterior) and one on the back (posterior).

When You're Using an AED:

• Make sure that no one is touching the person in cardiac arrest during the "analyze" or "shock" modes.

• Before applying the AED pads:

  ▶ Make sure the person's skin is dry before you apply the AED.

  ▶ If the person has a lot of chest hair, shave it off using a razor, if one is included with the AED, before you apply the AED pads. If there is no razor, you can take an extra set of pads, put them on the person's chest, and then pull them off to remove the hair.

  ▶ Remove any nitroglycerin, nicotine, or hormone patches that you see. Use gloves so that you don't absorb the medication through your hands.

• Check whether the person has an implanted pacemaker. Look on the chest for a small scar and a lump about the size of a matchbox. If the person has a pacemaker, apply the AED pads approximately 2.5 cm (1 in) away.

• If the person is lying in a puddle or other pool of water, do the "splash test." If you jump in the water and it splashes, it is deep enough to conduct an electric charge, so you must remove the person from the water before you use the AED.

CPR for a Baby

Check:

• Check the scene for danger.

• If it is safe to do so, check the baby.

Call:

• If the baby does not respond, have someone call EMS/9-1-1. If you are alone with a baby, do 5 cycles (two minutes) of CPR first, then take the baby with you (as long as you don't suspect a head or spine injury) to call EMS/9-1-1.

Care:

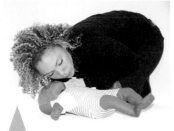

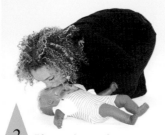

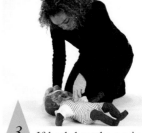

 1 Open the airway using the head-tilt/chin-lift and check for normal breathing for 5 to 10 seconds:

- Look, listen, and feel.

2 If you do not hear normal breathing, give two gentle breaths:

- Take a normal breath.
- Seal your lips tightly over the baby's mouth and nose.
- Give two gentle breaths. Each breath should last one second, with just enough volume to make the chest rise.

3 If both breaths go in, start CPR:

- Keep the airway open by using your hand to maintain a head-tilt.
- Place two fingers on the middle of the chest, just below the nipple line.
- Do 30 compressions. "Push hard, push fast."
- Allow the chest to recoil.
- Repeat cycles of compressions and breaths.

 4 Continue CPR until:

- More advanced care takes over.
- The scene becomes unsafe.
- You become physically unable to continue.

SPECIAL CONSIDERATIONS

 ### Air in the Stomach

Air in the stomach can make someone vomit. When an unconscious person vomits, the stomach contents may get into the lungs—a condition called *aspiration*. Aspiration makes giving rescue breaths more difficult, and it can be fatal.

Vomiting

In some situations a person may vomit while you are giving CPR.

If this happens:

1 Turn the person's head and body together as one unit onto the person's side, facing you.

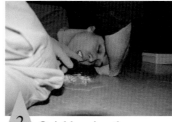

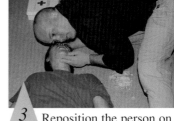

2 Quickly wipe the person's mouth clean.

3 Reposition the person on her back and continue with CPR.

Mouth-to-Nose Breathing

Sometimes you cannot seal your mouth well over the person's mouth to give rescue breaths because:

- The person's jaw or mouth is injured.

- The person's jaw or mouth is shut too tightly to open.

- Your mouth is too small to cover the person's mouth.

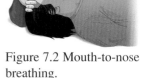

If this happens, breathe into the person's nose. (Figure 7.2) Block the mouth to stop air from escaping.

Figure 7.2 Mouth-to-nose breathing.

Mouth-to-Stoma Breathing

Some people have had an operation that removed part of their trachea. They breathe through an opening called a stoma in the front of the neck (Figure 7.3). Because air passes directly into the trachea through the stoma instead of through the mouth and nose, you should give rescue breaths into the stoma (Figure 7.4). Block the person's mouth and nose to stop air from escaping.

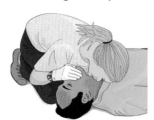

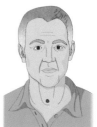

Figure 7.3 A stoma.

Figure 7.4 Mouth-to-stoma breathing.

One-Hand Compressions

If you have arthritis or your hands aren't strong enough for regular compressions, the one-hand compression method may work:

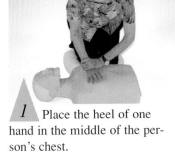

 1 Place the heel of one hand in the middle of the person's chest.

2 Grasp the wrist of the hand that is on the chest with your other hand.

3 Straighten your arms as much as possible without hurting yourself.

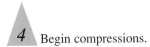 **4** Begin compressions.

CPR for a Pregnant Woman

- If a someone is available, ask her to find a soft object that you can place under the woman's right hip (Figure 7.5).

- Raising the right hip 7.5 to 10 cm (3 to 4 in) will help blood return to the heart. Do not interrupt CPR to find an object.

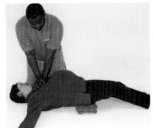

Figure 7.5 Place a soft object under the woman's right hip.

Adult	Child	Baby
Hand Position Two hands on the middle of the chest	**Hand Position** Two hands on the middle of the chest	**Hand Position** Two fingers on the middle of the chest (just below the nipple line)
Compress 4–5 cm (1.5–2 in)	**Compress** 1/3 to 1/2 of chest depth	**Compress** 1/3 to 1/2 of chest depth
Breathe Slowly until chest rises (1 second per breath)	**Breathe** Slowly until chest rises (1 second per breath)	**Breathe** Slowly until chest rises (1 second per gentle breath)
Cycle 30 compressions 2 breaths	**Cycle** 30 compressions 2 breaths	**Cycle** 30 compressions 2 gentle breaths

NOTES:

Additional Skills for Healthcare Providers

Additional Skills for Healthcare Providers

JAW THRUST

If you think the person might have a neck or back injury use a jaw thrust to open the airway instead of a head-tilt/chin-lift:

NOTE:

If you cannot keep the airway open with a jaw thrust, use the head-tilt/chin-lift. Remember, it is important to keep an open airway and get air in.

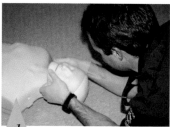

1 Place the fingers of both hands on the angles of the jaw.

2 Lift the jaw forward while keeping gentle pressure on the cheeks to keep the head from moving off the ground.

3 Place the mask over the person's mouth and nose.

4 Give two breaths. Each breath should last one second.

HOW TO DO A PULSE CHECK

▶ **Adult/Child**

During your ABC check, you can do a pulse check to check circulation. To check the carotid pulse of an adult or child:

NOTE:

The pulse may be hard to find if it is slow or weak. If after 10 seconds you are not absolutely certain there is a pulse, start CPR.

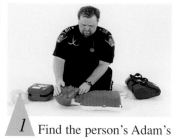

1 Find the person's Adam's apple.

2 Slide your fingers into the groove at the side of the neck closest to you.

NOTE:

If the pulse of an unresponsive child or baby is <60 beats per minute (bpm) and there are signs of poor perfusion (i.e., pallor cyanosis), begin chest compressions.

▶ Baby

To check the brachial pulse of a baby:

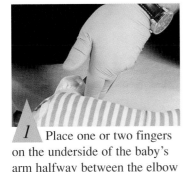

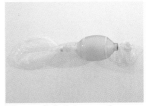

2 Push in against the upper arm bone gently. Keep your thumb off the arm.

1 Place one or two fingers on the underside of the baby's arm halfway between the elbow and the shoulder.

▶ Bag-Valve-Mask

- A Bag-Valve-Mask (BVM) has three parts: a bag, a valve, and a mask. They need to be put together before you can use the BVM (Figure 8.1).

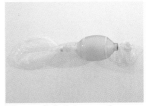

Figure 8.1 A bag-valve-mask.

- You need to have two rescuers to use a BVM:
  - ▶ One rescuer opens the injured person's airway with a head-tilt/chin-lift or jaw thrust and puts the mask on the person's face, making sure there is a tight seal.
  - ▶ The second rescuer squeezes the bag (Figure 8.2). Much like rescue breathing, the bag should be squeezed smoothly, not forcefully, just until the chest rises.

RESCUE BREATHING

First Aid for Respiratory Arrest

Adult or Child

Check:

- Check the scene for danger.
- If it is safe to do so, check the person.

Call:

- If the person does not respond, have someone call EMS/9-1-1 and get an AED if needed. If you are alone, call EMS/9-1-1 yourself and return to

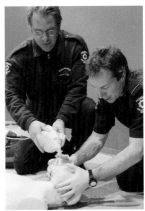

Figure 8.2 Ventilations with a BVM.

care for the person. If you are alone with a child, do one minute of rescue breathing first; then call EMS/9-1-1 and return to care for the child.

Care:

NOTE:

If the person is face down, roll the person over to assess breathing.

1 Open the airway and check for normal breathing for 5 to 10 seconds:

- Look, listen, and feel.

3 If both breaths go in, check for a carotid pulse for 10 seconds.

4 If there is a pulse, start rescue breathing:

- For an adult, give one breath every five to six seconds.
- For a child, give one breath every three to five seconds.

2 If you do not hear normal breathing, give two rescue breaths:

- Pinch the nose closed.
- Take a normal breath.
- Place the mask over the person's mouth and nose.
- Give two breaths. Each breath should last one second, with just enough volume to make the chest rise.

5 After two minutes of rescue breathing check again for signs of circulation and breathing for no more than 10 seconds:

- Look for movement, coughing, breathing, and colour of skin.
- Feel for a carotid pulse.

If there are signs of circulation and breathing, continue with secondary survey and continual care.

Secondary Survey:

Perform a secondary survey and treat any non-life-threatening injuries.

Continual Care:

Provide continual care.

If there are signs of circulation but no breathing:

Continue rescue breathing.

If there are no signs of circulation:

Do CPR.

Baby

Check:

- Check the scene for danger.
- If it is safe to do so, check the baby.

Call:

- If the baby does not respond, have someone call EMS/9-1-1. If you are alone with a baby, do one minute of rescue breathing first, then take the baby with you (as long as you don't suspect a head or spine injury) to call EMS/9-1-1.

Care:

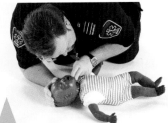

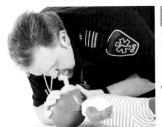

> **NOTE:**
> *Do not tilt the head back too far.*

1 Open the airway and check for normal breathing for 5 to 10 seconds:

- Look, listen, and feel.

2 If you do not hear normal breathing, give two rescue breaths:

- Place the mask over the baby's mouth and nose.
- Make sure there is a tight seal.
- Give two gentle breaths.

3 If both breaths go in, check for a brachial pulse.

4 If there is a pulse, start rescue breathing:

- Give the baby one breath every three to five seconds.

5 After two minutes of rescue breathing check again for signs of circulation and normal breathing for no more than 10 seconds:

- Look for movement, coughing, breathing, and colour of skin.
- Feel for a brachial pulse.

If there are signs of circulation and breathing, continue with secondary survey and continual care.

Secondary Survey:

Perform a secondary survey and treat any non-life-threatening injuries.

Continual Care:

Provide continual care.

If there are signs of circulation but no breathing:

Continue rescue breathing.

If there are no signs of circulation:

Do CPR.

A child is age one year to the onset of puberty for the purpose of all first aid, except when using an AED. In the case of AED, a child is age one to eight years old. For a child in this age range, use child pads. If the child is more than eight years old, adult electrode pads should be used. Follow the directions on the pads for placement.

If there is less than 2.5 cm (1 in) between the pads when on the chest, place one on the front of the chest (anterior) and one on the back (posterior).

 Unwitnessed Arrest

Performing CPR before applying the AED to a person whom you did not see go into arrest has been proven to be more beneficial than using an AED right away.

If you didn't see the cardiac arrest happen:

Check:

• Check the scene for danger.

• If it is safe to do so, check the person.

Call:

• If the person does not respond, have someone call EMS/9-1-1 and get an AED if one is available.

Care:

1. Confirm that the person is in arrest by checking breathing and circulation.

2. If there is no normal breathing, give two breaths.

3. If there are no signs of circulation, perform 5 cycles (two minutes) of CPR.

4. Follow the AED protocol.

▶ Two-Rescuer CPR/AED for an Adult or Child

Two rescuers can work together to give CPR to an adult or child:

1. One rescuer begins CPR while the second rescuer calls EMS/9-1-1 and gets an AED, if one is available.

2. When the second rescuer returns, one rescuer performs chest compressions while the other rescuer monitors the person's pulse to check whether the compressions are effective and gives rescue breaths/ventilations. Use the same technique and ratios as in adult CPR with one rescuer (30 compressions to 2 breaths/ventilations). For a child, if there are two rescuers, use a ratio of 15 compressions to 2 breaths/ventilations. Switch with the other rescuer every 2 minutes (between cycles) to maintain the quality of CPR.

▶ Two-Rescuer CPR for a Baby

Two rescuers can also work together to give CPR to a baby:

 1 One rescuer begins CPR while the second rescuer calls EMS/9-1-1.

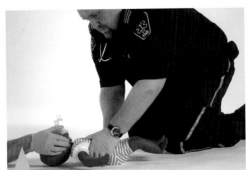

2 One rescuer encircles the baby's chest with both hands, spreading his fingers around the baby's back and placing both thumbs on the lower half of the baby's breastbone. The other rescuer monitors the baby's pulse to check whether the compressions are effective and gives rescue breaths/ventilations. For a baby, if there are two rescuers, use a ratio of 15 compressions to 2 breaths/ventilations.

NOTES:

Head and Spine Injuries

Head and Spine Injuries

An elderly woman is standing on a stepstool trying to reach the top shelf of a kitchen cupboard. She loses her balance and falls backwards, hitting her head on the counter as she falls.

Head and spine injuries can be fatal. People who survive can have physical difficulties and problems with how their brain works. This includes paralysis, speech and memory problems, and behavioural disorders. Head and spine injuries may lead to permanent disability.

HEAD AND SPINE INJURIES

▶ Causes of Head and Spine Injuries

- Motor vehicle collisions
- Falls
- Recreation and sports injuries
- Violent acts, such as assault

You should suspect that there are head and spine injuries in the following situations:

- A fall from any height
- Any diving injury
- A person found unconscious for unknown reasons
- Any injury that involves a strong blow to the head or trunk
- Any injury that causes a wound in the head or trunk
- A motor vehicle collision or roll-over or ejection from a vehicle
- Any injury in which the person's helmet is damaged
- A lightning strike
- Electrocution

As a First Aider, you may not be able to determine how much damage has taken place without advanced medical assessment and diagnosis, so always treat the injury as if it were serious.

▶ Preventing Head and Spine Injuries

- Always buckle up. Wear safety belts and shoulder restraints when you're in a car.

- Babies and children should always ride in approved safety seats. Make sure the seat is designed for the child's age and weight and make sure it is properly installed.

- For any activities for which you need protection, wear a properly fitting helmet approved by the Canadian Standards Association (CSA), proper eyewear, and other protective equipment. Helmets should fit comfortably and securely. All bicycle riders—adults, teens, and children—should wear a helmet.

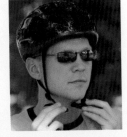

- Take safety precautions in all contact sports by wearing proper protection, such as mouthpieces, helmets, and eyewear.

- Never join in a new sport without knowing the rules and risks involved.

- Prevent falls around the home and workplace with non-slip floors, non-slip treads on stairs, handrails on staircases, rugs secured with double-sided adhesive tape, and handrails by the bathtub and toilet when necessary.

- Make sure that there is good lighting in stairways and hallways.

- If there are small children in your home, put gates at the top and bottom of the stairways.

- Make sure your workplace is clean and tidy. Keep floors and aisles uncluttered and make sure there is nothing blocking stairways, work sites, or exits.

- Drink responsibly. Alcohol is often a factor in serious motor vehicle collisions and water injuries. Alcohol slows down your reflexes and gives you a false feeling of confidence.

- Prescription drugs and common drugstore medications can also make driving or operating machinery dangerous, so follow the directions on the package carefully.

- Check equipment, such as warehouse forklifts, ladders, and scaffolding, regularly for worn or loose parts.
- Use ladders carefully and correctly.
- Always be very careful around water:
  ▶ Before you dive, make sure the water is deep enough. Pools at homes, motels, or hotels may not be safe for diving.
  ▶ Enter unknown water feet first.
  ▶ Enter above-ground pools feet first.
  ▶ Always swim with a buddy.
  ▶ Before diving, check for objects below the surface, such as logs or pilings.
  ▶ When you're bodysurfing, keep your arms in front of you to protect your head and neck.

▶ Signs and Symptoms of Head Injuries

- Changes in level of consciousness and behaviour
- Severe pain or pressure in the head
- Blood or clear fluid coming from the ears or nose
- Heavy bleeding from the head
- Unusual bumps on the head
- Seizures
- Problems breathing or seeing properly
- Nausea or vomiting
- Unequal pupil size
- A headache that won't go away
- Weakness or an inability to use a leg or arm
- Loss of balance
- Bruising of the head, especially around the eyes and behind the ears

These signs and symptoms alone do not always mean a serious head injury. However, you should always call EMS/9-1-1 when you suspect that there may be a serious head or spine injury.

Bleeding inside the skull can happen slowly, so the symptoms may take time to appear.

First Aid for Head Injuries

Whenever you suspect that there might be a head injury:

Check:

- Check the scene for danger.

- If it is safe to do so, approach the person. Tell the person not to move. Make sure that your movements won't make the person's head or neck move. Then check the person.

Call:

- Have someone call EMS/9-1-1. If you are alone, call EMS/9-1-1 yourself, then return to care for the person.

Care:

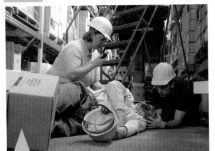

> **NOTE:**
> *Remember your gloves and other barrier devices.*

2 If the person is wearing a helmet, leave it on unless it makes it difficult for you to manage the ABCs.

1 Once you reach the person, make sure the head and spine move as little as possible by placing your hands on both sides of the person's head. Gently support the person's head in the position in which you found it until EMS personnel arrive.

3 If the ABCs are present, perform a secondary survey as best as you can without letting go of the head. If there is another First Aider or bystander, have him help you.

Secondary Survey:

Perform a secondary survey and treat any non-life-threatening injuries.

Continual Care:

Provide continual care until EMS personnel arrive.

Leave the person in the position he was found, unless the person is in immediate danger or has life-threatening injuries that need immediate attention.

Any injury that is serious enough to fracture or dislocate the jaw, nose, or other facial bones can cause other head or spine injuries.

CONCUSSION

A *concussion* happens when a blow to the head shakes the brain inside the skull. This can result in bleeding and/or swelling in or around the brain.

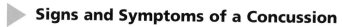 **Signs and Symptoms of a Concussion**

- In most cases, if someone loses consciousness, it is for only a short period of time, although sometimes it lasts several minutes.

- The person may say that he "blacked out" or "saw stars."

- Sometimes the person is confused or has memory loss.

 First Aid for a Concussion

See "First Aid for Head Injuries."

> **NOTE:**
>
> *The Canadian Red Cross offers a series of violence prevention education programs for adults, youth, and children through our RespectED: Violence and Abuse Prevention program.*

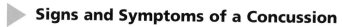 **Shaken Baby Syndrome**

When a baby won't stop crying, some people get so angry and frustrated that they shake the baby. This can cause fractures, heavy bleeding, bruising, and brain swelling, which stops oxygen from getting to the brain. Seek medical attention immediately.

Never shake a baby or a child, no matter what. Place the baby on its back in a safe place and let it cry while you take a few deep breaths and then try again to soothe the baby.

Contact your local help or crisis line if you need help to deal with anger or frustration.

 First Aid for a Scalp Injury

Check:

- Check the scene for danger.

- If it is safe to do so, check the person.

Call:

- Call EMS/9-1-1 if you are not sure how serious a scalp injury is or if you feel a dip, a soft area, or pieces of bone.

Care:

- Make sure ABCs are present.

Secondary Survey:

Perform a secondary survey and treat any non-life-threatening injuries. Pay particular attention to the area of injury because hair may be hiding part of the wound.

If there doesn't seem to be a fracture:

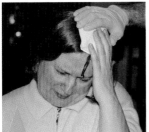

2 Secure the dressings with a bandage.

1 Put dressings on the wound and have the person hold them in place with her hand to control the bleeding.

If you feel a dip, a soft area, or pieces of bone:

1. Treat the injury as a head injury.

2. Put direct pressure on the wound only if the bleeding is severe.

3. Try to control the bleeding with pressure on the area around the wound.

Continual Care:

Provide continual care until EMS personnel arrive.

▶ **Signs and Symptoms of Spine Injuries**

- Changes in level of consciousness and behaviour

- Severe pain or pressure in the neck or back

- Numbness, tingling, or loss of feeling in any body part

- Unusually positioned neck or back

- Heavy bleeding from the neck or back

- Seizures
- Loss of bladder or bowel control

- Problems breathing
- Shock

These signs and symptoms alone do not always mean a serious spine injury. However, you should always call EMS/9-1-1 when you suspect that there may be a serious head or spine injury.

 ## First Aid for Spine Injuries

Whenever you suspect that there might be a spine injury:

Check:

- Check the scene for danger.

- If it is safe to do so, approach the person. Tell the person not to move. Make sure that your movements won't make the person's head or neck move. Then check the person.

Call:

- Have someone call EMS/9-1-1. If you are alone, call EMS/9-1-1 yourself, then return to care for the person.

Care:

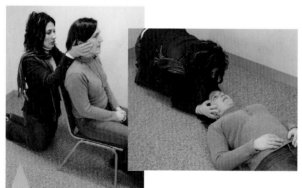

> **NOTE:**
> *Remember your gloves and other barrier devices.*

1 Once you reach the person, make sure the head and spine move as little as possible by placing your hands on both sides of the person's head. Gently support the person's head in the position in which you found it until EMS personnel arrive.

2 If the person is wearing a helmet, leave it on unless it makes it difficult for you to manage the ABCs.

Secondary Survey:

Perform a secondary survey as best as you can without letting go of the head. If there is another First Aider or bystander, have him help you. Treat any non-life-threatening injuries.

Continual Care:

Provide continual care until EMS personnel arrive.

> A person who has no signs or symptoms may still have a spine injury. If the cause of the injury means that a head or spine injury is likely, treat the person as if she has one.

▶ Moving a Person With a Head or Spine Injury

A log roll (Figure 9.1) is the safest way to move a person with a head or spine injury. You should do this if:

- You need to clear the person's airway.

- You suspect a life-threatening injury on the back.

- You need to move the person onto something to move them from a dangerous situation.

Figure 9.1 A log roll.

Unless you have the proper equipment and training, wait for EMS personnel to arrive.

▶ Modified H.A.IN.E.S. Recovery Position

The modified H.A.IN.E.S. Recovery Position is to be used only if an unconscious person who has a suspected spinal injury must be left alone.

Starting with the person on their back:

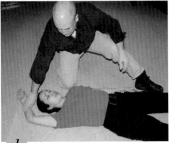 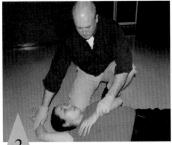 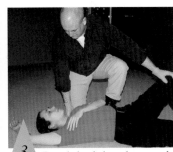

1 Kneel beside the injured person's waist. Raise the person's arm furthest away from you by rotating it outwards, while keeping the palm facing upwards.

2 Place the arm nearest to you across the chest, with fingers pointing to the opposite shoulder.

3 Bend the injured person's nearest lower leg at the knee.

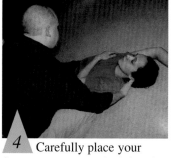

4 Carefully place your forearm nearest to the injured person's head and neck, under the nearest shoulder to provide extra leverage, and to avoid pushing on the head and neck. Place the hand near the head under the hollow of the injured person's neck and head to provide stabilization. DO NOT push or lift the head or neck.

NOTE:

Ensure the head remains in contact with the injured person's raised arm and supported by your hand.

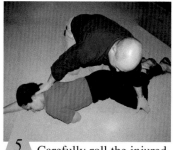

5 Carefully roll the injured person away from yourself, by simultaneously pushing on the nearest shoulder, with the forearm of your stabilizing hand, and the flexed knee.

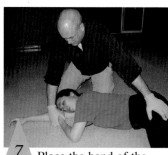

7 Place the hand of the person's upper arm on the outstretched arm against the forehead.

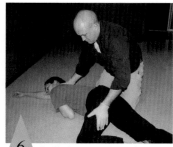

6 Pull the near leg closer to the chest.

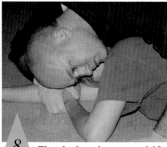

8 Check the airway and if required, clear with the face turned slightly downwards to permit drainage from the mouth.

Bone, Muscle, and Joint Injuries

Bone, Muscle, and Joint Injuries

A roofer is carrying a box of tools across the building site. He trips on a pile of lumber and falls forward, spraining his ankle and breaking a wrist.

BONE, MUSCLE, AND JOINT INJURIES

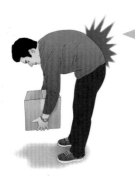

Strain – the stretching or tearing of muscles or tendons.

Sprain – the stretching or tearing of ligaments at a joint.

Dislocation – an injury that moves a bone out of its normal position at a joint.

Fracture – a break, chip, or crack in a bone. In an open fracture, the bone breaks through the skin; in a closed fracture, the skin isn't broken.

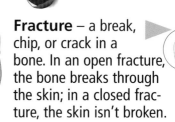

▶ Causes of Bone, Muscle, and Joint Injuries

Bone, muscle, and joint injuries can occur in many ways. The causes include:

- Falls
- Awkward or sudden movements
- Motor vehicle collisions

- A direct blow to the body
- Repetitive forces, such as running (stress fractures)
- Many contact and non-contact sports

▶ Preventing Bone, Muscle, and Joint Injuries

- Always wear seat belts and shoulder restraints when you're in a vehicle.
- Small children must be in approved and properly installed child restraint systems (car seats, booster seats).
- During activities, wear the appropriate safety equipment (such as helmets, goggles, and pads).
- When you are bicycling, always wear an approved bicycle helmet.
- Put non-slip adhesive or mat in the bath.
- Wear proper protection when you're playing contact sports.
- Know the risks and rules of new sports.
- Check the water depth before diving.
- Enter above-ground pools feet first.
- Stretch before exercising.
- Know your limits. When you are too tired or frustrated, take a break.

▶ Signs and Symptoms of Bone, Muscle, and Joint Injuries

- Pain
- Deformity or a broken bone sticking out of the skin
- Swelling
- Bruising
- Inability to move the body part or difficulty moving it
- The sound of a snap or pop when the injury happened
- Shock

First Aid for Bone, Muscle, and Joint Injuries

Check:

- Check the scene for danger.
- If it is safe to do so, check the person.

Call:

- Call EMS/9-1-1 if there is a problem with the ABCs or if the person needs transportation.

You should call EMS/9-1-1 when:

- The injury involves the head, neck, or back.
- The injury makes walking difficult.
- You suspect that there may be more than one injury.
- There are injuries to the thigh bone or pelvis.
- There is an altered level of consciousness.

Care:

- Make sure ABCs are present.

NOTE:	Secondary Survey:
If you expect the ambulance will arrive in a few minutes, keep the person still and do not splint the injury. If the ambulance is going to take longer to arrive, immobilize the injury in the position found, using bandages, slings, splints, or blankets, if it does not cause further damage or pain.	Perform a secondary survey and treat any non-life-threatening injuries:

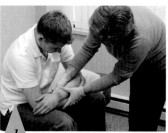

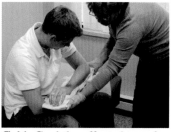

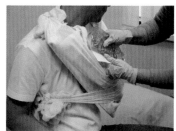

1 Treat the injury using the RICE method:

Rest: Have the person stop what he was doing.

Immobilize: Immobilize the injured area in the position that you found it.

Cold: Cool the affected area for 20 minutes of every hour for the first 24 to 48 hours. If you use ice, put some sort of thin cloth or pad between it and the bare skin to avoid freezing the skin.

Elevate: Keep the injured area above the level of the heart if possible. However, do not raise the injured area if moving it will cause pain.

R - **Rest**

I - **Immobilize**

C - **Cold**

E - **Elevate**

Continual Care:

Provide continual care.

Splinting Guidelines

There are four types of splints:

- **Soft splints** include folded blankets, towels, pillows, and bandages.

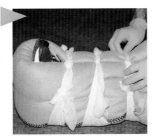

- **Rigid splints** immobilize an injured body part by securing it to something rigid, such as a board, a rolled newspaper, a tree branch, etc.

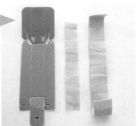

- **Anatomical splints** use another body part for support. For example, you could immobilize an injured leg by securing it to the uninjured leg.

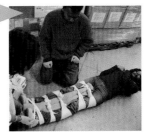

- **Slings** are looped around the neck to support an arm, hand, or wrist.

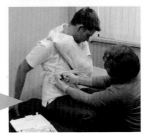

No matter what type of splint you use, follow these steps:

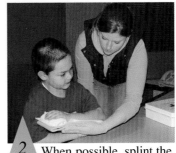

1 Check for skin temperature and colour below the injured area before and after splinting. The area should be warm, indicating good circulation. If the area is cold before splinting, seek medical attention quickly. If the area was warm before splinting and cold afterwards, the splint may be too tight. Loosen it gently.

2 When possible, splint the injured part in the position in which it was found.

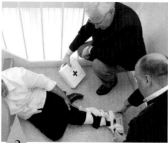

3 For joint injuries, splint the bone above and below the site of the injury.

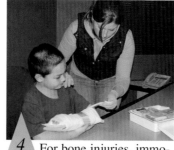

4 For bone injuries, immobilize joints above and below the site of the injury.

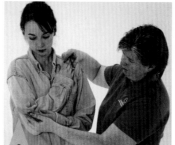

5 Always pad a rigid or anatomical splint to make the person more comfortable.

Applying a tube sling for a collarbone fracture:

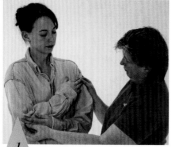

1 Check circulation by checking the fingers for warmth and colour compared to the other limb.

- Remove any rings the person is wearing.
- Ask the person if they have any numbness or tingling in the fingers.

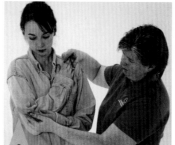

2 Put the forearm of the injured side across the chest, with fingers pointing at the opposite arm.

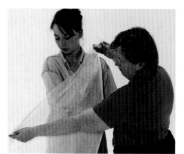

- Position the open triangular bandage over the forearm and hand.
- The point of the triangular bandage should extend past the elbow and shoulder.

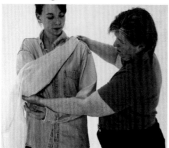

- Support the forearm and carefully tuck the bandage under all the way from the hand to the elbow.

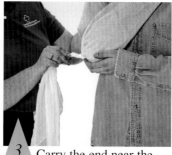

3 Carry the end near the elbow around the back.

- Twist the top of the point of the bandage near the elbow to secure the elbow from coming out of the sling.

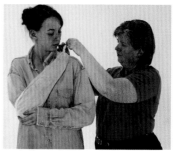

- Adjust the height of the sling to make sure it is supporting the arm.
- Tie the ends together in the hollow of the neck on the uninjured side.

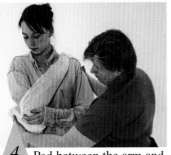

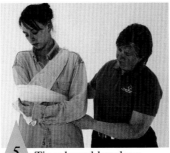

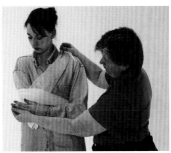

4 Pad between the arm and the body, in the natural hollow, with soft, firm material.

5 Tie a broad bandage from the elbow on the injured side across the body.

Check circulation again for colour or warmth.

- Ask the person if they have any numbness or tingling in the fingers.

If fingers are bluish or cold or if the person feels numbness and tingling loosen the bandages. If loosening the bandages does not improve circulation call EMS/9-1-1 immediately.

- Slings should fit tight enough to restrict movement, but not so tight that blood flow is affected.

OSTEOPOROSIS

Osteoporosis is a leading cause of bone and joint injuries in older people. It happens when the amount of calcium in your bones decreases, making the bones frail. It is not usually discovered until after age 65, but it can begin at a very early age. Osteoporosis affects one in four women, but it is less common in men.

▶ Preventing Osteoporosis

- Build strong bones at an early age.
- Make sure you get enough calcium.
- Make sure you get enough vitamin D (your body needs vitamin D so that it can absorb calcium).
- Exercise regularly.

Talk to your doctor about testing and treatment for osteoporosis.

▶ Signs and Symptoms of Osteoporosis

- Fractures occur with little or no external force.
- Fractures of the hips, vertebrae, and wrists are particularly common.

NOTE:

Often, osteoporosis is not diagnosed until after a fracture occurs.

NOTES:

Wound Care

Wound Care

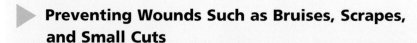

On a camping trip, your four-year-old daughter trips and lands in the bright red embers of the campfire. You hear her crying and turn to see burns on the child's hands and arms, as well as a large splinter of wood sticking out of one hand.

Wounds such as bruises, scrapes, and small cuts are very common injuries. There are many ways to cause these types of wounds.

> ### Preventing Wounds Such as Bruises, Scrapes, and Small Cuts

- Develop safe play habits to prevent injury, such as not running with sharp objects.
- Use helmets, knee pads, and elbow pads during sports and when using sports equipment such as bikes, skateboards, and in-line skates.
- Wear proper safety equipment in the workplace.

BRUISES

A *bruise* is a discoloured area of the skin that is created when blood and other fluids seep into nearby tissues (Figure 11.1).

> ### Causes of Bruises

- Some kind of blow or impact to the body

> ### Signs and Symptoms of Bruises

- Discolouring (red, purple, black, or blue areas)
- Swelling
- Pain

Figure 11.1 A bruise.

First Aid for Bruises

Check:

- Check the scene for danger.

• If it is safe to do so, check the person.

Call:

• Call EMS/9-1-1 if you suspect there may be more serious injuries.

Care:

• Make sure ABCs are present.

Secondary Survey:

Perform a secondary survey and treat any non-life-threatening injuries:

1. Cool the area to help reduce pain and swelling.

2. When you cool the area, put some sort of cloth or pad between the ice and the skin.

Continual Care:

Apply the ice for 20 minutes of every hour for as long as the person keeps feeling pain. Place a cloth between the ice and the person's skin.

> If a person feels severe pain or cannot move a body part without pain, or if you think the force that caused the injury was great enough to cause serious damage or severe bleeding, call EMS/9-1-1 immediately. You may be dealing with internal bleeding, head or spine injuries, or bone, muscle, and joint injuries. See the previous chapters for instructions on how to care for these injuries.

CUTS & SCRAPES

A *cut* is a wound where the skin has been split open or torn away. The edges of the wound can be jagged or smooth (Figure 11.2).

Scrapes are wounds where the skin has been rubbed or scraped away (Figure 11.3).

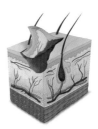
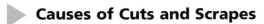

Figure 11.2 A cut.

▶ **Causes of Cuts and Scrapes**

• Any action that rubs or scrapes the skin away

• A sharp object

▶ **Signs and Symptoms of Cuts and Scrapes**

• Possible bleeding

• Pain

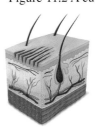
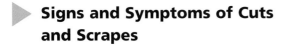

Figure 11.3 A scrape.

First Aid for Cuts and Scrapes

Check:

• Check the scene for danger.

• If it is safe to do so, check the person.

Call:

• Call EMS/9-1-1 if you suspect that there may be more serious injuries.

Care:

• Make sure ABCs are present.

Secondary Survey:

Perform a secondary survey and treat any non-life-threatening injuries:

> **NOTE:**
>
> *Remember your gloves and other barrier devices.*

1 Use non-latex gloves. If non-latex gloves are not available, use some other kind of barrier between your hand and the wound. If possible, have the injured person use her own hand.

There is usually minimal bleeding with scrapes. If this is the case, go directly to step 2. If there is bleeding, put direct pressure on the wound until it stops.

2 Wash the wound thoroughly with soap and water.

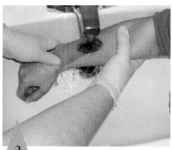

3 If possible, rinse the wound for five minutes with clean, running tap water.

4 If an antibiotic ointment or cream is available, put it on the wound as recommended by a pharmacist. Ask the person if he has a sensitivity to any antibiotics, such as penicillin. If so, do not apply the ointment.

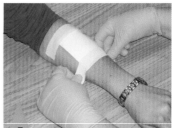

5 Cover the wound with a sterile dressing and/or bandage.

Continual Care:

Watch for signs of infection. (See the section on infection on page 117.)

If there is a great deal of dirt or contamination in the wound, the injured person should seek medical attention.

If the blood soaks through the dressings, add more dressings on top. Do not remove the soaked dressings that are in direct contact with the wound! If you cannot control the bleeding, make sure the person gets medical attention immediately.

 A Stitch in Time

Wounds should be stitched by a trained medical professional in the first few hours after an injury. A wound may require stitching if:

- The edges of the skin do not fall together

- The wound is more than 2.5 cm (1 in) long

- The wound is near joints on the hands or feet

- The wound is on the face

Stitches will help:

- Speed up healing

- Reduce the chance of infection

- Leave a less noticeable scar

PUNCTURE WOUNDS

A *puncture wound* happens when something pointed creates a hole in the skin (Figure 11.4).

 Causes of Puncture Wounds

- Injuries from pointed objects such as nails or pieces of glass

- Animal bites

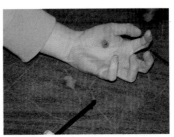

Figure 11.4 A puncture wound.

▶ Preventing puncture wounds

- Develop safe play habits to prevent injury, such as not running with sharp objects.

- Wear proper safety equipment in the workplace.

- Stay away from animals you are unfamiliar with.

- Wear shoes when walking outside.

- Always sweep up broken glass right away. Remove nails from boards and dispose of them properly.

▶ Signs and Symptoms of Puncture Wounds

- Minimal external bleeding

- Possible bruising

- A hole where the object went through the skin

▣ First Aid for Puncture Wounds

Check:

- Check the scene for danger.

- If it is safe to do, check the person.

Call:

- Call EMS/9-1-1 if the wound is deep or large.

Care:

- Make sure ABCs are present.

Secondary Survey:

Perform a secondary survey and treat any non-life-threatening injuries:

NOTE:

Remember your gloves and other barrier devices.

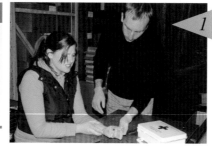

 Use non-latex gloves. If non-latex gloves are not available, use some other kind of barrier between your hand and the wound. If possible, have the injured person use her own hand.

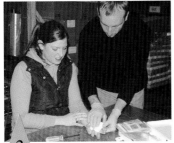

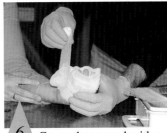

△ **2** If there is much bleeding, put direct pressure on the wound until it stops.

△ **3** Once the bleeding is controlled and there is no risk of causing more bleeding, wash the wound thoroughly with soap and water.

△ **4** If possible, rinse the wound for five minutes with clean, running tap water.

△ **5** If an antibiotic ointment or cream is available, put it on the wound as recommended by a pharmacist. Ask the person if she has a sensitivity to any antibiotics, such as penicillin. If so, do not apply the ointment.

△ **6** Cover the wound with a sterile dressing and/or bandage.

Continual Care:

Watch for signs of infection. (See the section on infection on page 117.)

▶ **Dressings and Bandages**

Dressings are pads you put on an open wound to absorb blood and other fluids and to prevent infection. *Bandages* are materials you can use to wrap or cover a dressing. They are used to control bleeding, to apply pressure, to provide support, or to protect a wound from dirt and infection.

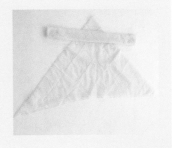

If a bandage is put on too tightly, the limb below the bandage may become cold or numb or begin to turn blue or paler than normal. If this happens, loosen the bandage.

If blood soaks through the bandage, use more dressings and another bandage. The dressing in contact with the wound should remain in place.

IMPALED OBJECTS

If the object that created the injury is stuck in the wound, it's called an *impaled object* (Figure 11.5).

▶ **Causes of Impaled Objects**

- Any force that causes an object to penetrate the skin and underlying tissues.

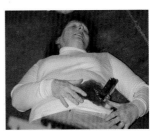

Figure 11.5 An impaled object.

Preventing Impaled Objects

- See "Preventing Puncture Wounds."

 Signs and Symptoms of Impaled Objects

- An object sticking out of the body
- Pain
- Shock
- Bleeding

 First Aid for Impaled Objects

Check:

- Check the scene for danger.
- If it is safe to do so, check the person.

LOOK OUT FOR:

If the impaled object is a weapon, ensure that the scene is safe.

Call:

- Call EMS/9-1-1 if the impaled object is large or if it is impaled in the head, neck, or torso.

Care:

- Make sure ABCs are present.

Secondary Survey:

Perform a secondary survey and treat any non-life-threatening injuries:

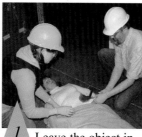
1 Leave the object in place.

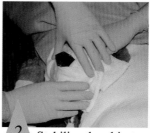
2 Stabilize the object by putting bulky dressings around it.

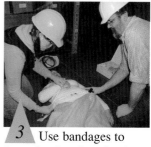
3 Use bandages to keep the dressings in place.

NOTE:

If the object is impaled in the head, treat the injury as a head injury (see Chapter 9).

Continual Care:

Make sure the person gets medical attention.

NOSEBLEEDS

▶ Causes of Nosebleeds

- Forceful nose blowing
- Trauma to the nose
- Dry weather conditions
- High blood pressure
- Bleeding disorders

▶ Preventing Nosebleeds

- Use a humidifier if the air indoors is dry.
- Wear protective athletic equipment when participating in sports that could cause injury to the nose.
- Encourage gentle nose blowing.

▶ Signs and Symptoms of Nosebleeds

- Blood coming from the nose

 ### First Aid for Nosebleeds

Check:

- Check the scene for danger.
- If it is safe to do so, check the person.

Call:

- Call EMS/9-1-1 if the person loses consciousness, if the bleeding continues after 15 minutes, if the bleeding starts again, or if the bleeding was caused as a result of a medical condition or head injury.

Care:

- Make sure ABCs are present.

Secondary Survey:

Perform a secondary survey and treat any non-life-threatening injuries:

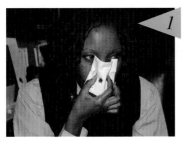

1 Have the person sit with the head slightly forward while pinching the nostrils for 10 to 15 minutes.

> **NOTE:**
> *Remember your gloves and other barrier devices.*

2 Once you have controlled the bleeding, tell the person to avoid rubbing, blowing, or picking the nose because this could start the bleeding again.

3 If the person loses consciousness, place her in the recovery position to allow blood to drain from the nose.

4 If the bleed was caused by an object in the nose and the object is easy to grab, then gently pull it out. However, don't feel around inside the nostril with your finger. If there is an object in the nose that you cannot remove easily, the person should seek medical attention.

If the nosebleed was caused by a severe head injury, do not pinch the nose.

Continual Care:

Later, have the person rub a little water-soluble jelly inside the nostril to help keep it from drying out.

KNOCKED-OUT TEETH

Causes of Knocked-Out Teeth

• Any kind of blow or fall that involves the mouth

Preventing Knocked-Out Teeth

• Wear appropriate equipment when playing sports, such as a mouth-guard or face mask.

• Always wear a seat belt while in the car and do not eat or drink in a moving car.

Signs and Symptoms of Knocked-Out Teeth

• Missing tooth, usually from some kind of impact

• Bleeding (although this is often very minimal)

• Pain in the mouth

 ### First Aid for Knocked-Out Teeth

Check:

• Check the scene for danger.

• If it is safe to do so, check the person.

Call:

- Call EMS/9-1-1 if the knocked-out tooth was caused by a forceful blow to the head, the person was knocked unconscious, or you suspect that there may be other more serious injuries.

Care:

- Make sure ABCs are present.

Because a knocked-out tooth is often caused by an impact, the person may also have airway problems (see Chapter 5) or head and spine injuries (see Chapter 9).

Secondary Survey:

Perform a secondary survey and treat any non-life-threatening injuries:

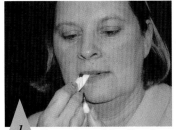 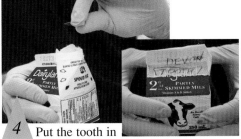

1 Control any bleeding by having the person bite down on a sterile or clean dressing.

2 Carefully pick up the tooth by the crown (the white part), not the root.

3 Gently rinse off the tooth in water. Do not scrub it or remove any tissue fragments that are attached.

4 Put the tooth in milk, if possible, or in water and keep it with the person. If there is no milk or water, wrap the tooth in a clean cloth or gauze. Seal the container with tape and label it with the name of the person, date, and time.

5 Get the person to a dentist as soon as possible. The greatest chance for repair is during the first hour after the tooth was knocked out.

Continual Care:

Provide continual care.

EYE INJURIES

▶ Causes of Eye Injuries

- Foreign objects or particles in the eye
- Impact to the eye
- Radiation or burns

▶ Preventing Eye and Ear Injuries

- Wear appropriate equipment in the workplace (such as a hard hat, ear plugs, or safety glasses/face shields).
- Wear appropriate equipment when you are playing sports. (For example, wear a batting helmet when you are playing baseball.)
- Get trained on all equipment at your workplace that might be dangerous.
- Wear proper protection when using loud equipment such as lawn mowers and chainsaws.

▶ Signs and Symptoms of Eye Injuries

- Pain and irritation in the eye
- Difficulty opening the eye
- Watering of the eye
- Redness
- Problems seeing properly
- Deformities

First Aid for Eye Injuries

Check:

- Check the scene for danger.
- If it is safe to do so, check the person.

Call:

- Call EMS/9-1-1 if you suspect that there may be a head or spine injury, if there is an impaled object in or near the eye, or if the eye is out of the socket.

Care:

- Make sure ABCs are present.

> **NOTE:**
> *Remember your gloves and other barrier devices.*

Injuries to the eyeball are very serious and require special care. Never put direct pressure on the eyeball.

Secondary Survey:

Perform a secondary survey and treat any non-life-threatening injuries:

If there is a **foreign object** in the eye but it is not impaled:

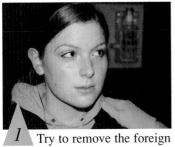 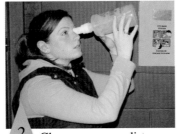

1 Try to remove the foreign object by having the person blink several times. The eye will produce tears that may wash it out.

2 Clean away any dirt around the eye and then gently flush the eye with water (away from the unaffected eye).

Continual Care:

If the object remains in the eye, the person should seek medical attention.

If there is an **impaled object** in the eye:

1 Have the person rest comfortably.

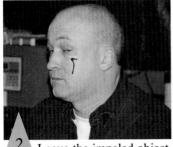 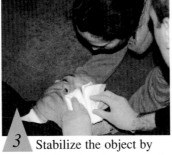 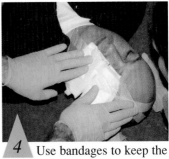

2 Leave the impaled object in the eye.

3 Stabilize the object by putting bulky dressings around it and being careful not to put pressure on the eye.

4 Use bandages to keep the dressings in place.

Flash burn

If the eyes were **flash burned** (from welding, for example):

1. Cover the eyes with a cool, wet cloth.

2. Make sure the person gets medical attention.

Any wound near the eye should be treated as an eye injury.

EAR INJURIES

▶ Causes of Ear Injuries

* Impact
* Head injury
* Foreign objects or substances in the ear
* Cuts or tears
* Loud noise

▶ Signs and Symptoms of Ear Injuries

* Blood or other fluid from within the ear
* Sudden or intense pain in the ear
* Hearing problems
* Swelling or deformity

First Aid for Ear Injuries

Check:

* Check the scene for danger.
* If it is safe to do so, check the person.

Call:

* Call EMS/9-1-1 if there is blood or other fluid draining from the ear.

Care:

* Make sure ABCs are present.

If the ear injury is the result of an explosion or a diving injury, call EMS/9-1-1.

Secondary Survey:

Perform a secondary survey and treat any non-life-threatening injuries.

If the bleeding is from an **external wound:**

1. Treat it the same way you would treat any other wound.

If there is a **foreign object** in the ear, you don't suspect a head or spine injury, and the object looks like it can easily be removed:

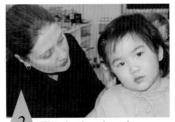

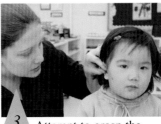

 1 Pull down on the ear lobe.

2 Tilt the head to the affected side. Gently shake the head to remove the object.

3 Attempt to grasp the object and pull it out.

If the person has a **serious head or spine injury** and **blood or other fluid is in the ear canal or draining from the ear:**

1. Let the ear drain. Do not apply direct pressure. Do not move the person if possible.

2. Cover it lightly with a sterile dressing.

Continual Care:

Provide continual care until EMS personnel arrive.

INFECTION

An *infection* is a condition caused by the invasion of the body by germs (Figure 11.6).

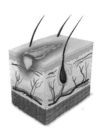

Figure 11.6 An infection.

▶ **Causes of Infection**

• Dirt, foreign bodies, or other things containing germs that get in a wound

▶ **Preventing Infection**

• Always wash your hands after giving first aid.

• Whenever possible, wear gloves if you will be coming in contact with someone's body fluids.

• Whenever possible, use sterile dressings when you are caring for wounds.

• Keep your immunizations up to date. If you have been wounded and have not received a tetanus shot in more than five years, seek medical attention.

• Use antibiotic ointment on a wound to help reduce the risk of infection.

• Keep the wound area clean and wash regularly.

Signs and Symptoms of Infection

- Redness
- Pus
- Tenderness
- Swelling

- Red streaks moving away from the wound
- Heat or warmth
- Fever

AMPUTATIONS

An *amputation* is a complete or partial severing of a body part (Figure 11.7). Although there is a lot of damage to the tissues, bleeding is usually not severe.

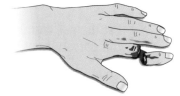

Figure 11.7 An amputation.

 Causes of Amputations

- Any force great enough to completely or partially cut or tear away a limb from the rest of the body

 Preventing Amputations

- Wear proper equipment when working around machinery.
- Follow the manufacturer's instructions when you are using equipment at the workplace or in the home.

 Signs and Symptoms of Amputations

- Shock
- Pain
- A part of the body completely or partially disconnected from the rest of the body
- Bleeding

First Aid for Amputations

Check:

- Check the scene for danger.
- If it is safe to do so, check the person.

Call:

- Have someone call EMS/9-1-1. If you are alone, call EMS/9-1-1 yourself, then return to care for the person.

Care:

- Make sure ABCs are present.

Secondary Survey:

Perform a secondary survey and treat any non-life-threatening injuries:

1 Treat any bleeding with direct pressure.

2 Try to retrieve the amputated body part.

3 Wrap the amputated part in a clean cloth or gauze.

4 Place the amputated part in a plastic bag.

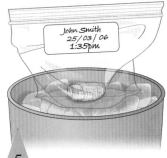

5 Keep the amputated part cool by placing the bag on ice and wrap it so that the body part does not freeze.

6 Label the container that contains the body part (person's name, date, and time).

7 Make sure the amputated part goes with the injured person to the hospital.

> **NOTE:**
>
> *If the limb is partially disconnected from the body, put the limb back in place and treat the injury as an open wound or fracture.*

Continual Care:

Provide continual care until EMS personnel arrive.

CRUSH INJURIES

A **crush injury** occurs when there is a great deal of pressure on a part of the body. It is often caused by being squeezed between two heavy or immobile objects (Figure 11.8).

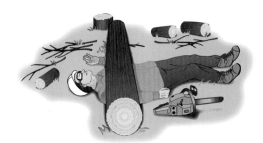

Figure 11.8 A crush injury.

Preventing Crush Injuries

- Be familiar with your surroundings.
- Be familiar with your equipment and get trained in its proper use.
- Make sure your equipment is in good, safe, working order.
- Wear protective gear.
- Stay alert.

Signs and Symptoms of a Crush Injury

- Person may still be crushed under the object(s) or between two objects
- Possible wound
- Shock
- Deformity
- Pain
- Signs of internal bleeding

First Aid for a Crush Injury

NOTE:

Remove the object only if you can do it safely, without causing any further harm.

Check:

- Check the scene for danger.
- If it is safe to do so, check the person.

Call:

- Have someone call EMS/9-1-1. If you are alone, call EMS/9-1-1 yourself, then return to care for the person.

NOTE:

If the object is crushing the person's head, neck, chest, or abdomen, or the person cannot breathe, remove it immediately. If it is crushing another body part, leave the object where it is until EMS personnel arrive.

Care:

- Make sure ABCs are present.

Secondary Survey:

Perform a secondary survey and treat any non-life-threatening injuries.

Continual Care:

Provide continual care until EMS personnel arrive.

PENETRATING CHEST INJURIES

Chest injuries can cause a breathing emergency if the lungs are punctured by a penetrating object. A puncture that goes through the rib cage may let air or blood into the chest through the wound (Figure 11.9).

► Causes of Penetrating Chest Injuries

• Weapons, such as knives or guns

• Falls onto objects

• Industrial incidents

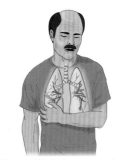

Figure 11.9 A penetrating chest injury.

• Other penetrating forces that create a wound in the chest wall

► Preventing Penetrating Chest Injuries

Chest injuries can often be prevented by good safety practices in all areas of life, including:

• Driving motor vehicles
• Working around the home

• Sports
• Occupational activities

• Recreational activities

Follow the safety guidelines throughout this manual for preventing injuries.

► Signs and Symptoms of Penetrating Chest Injuries

• Difficulty breathing

• Bleeding from an open chest wound (Figure 11.10)

• A sucking sound coming from the wound with each breath

• Severe pain at the site of the injury

• Coughing up blood

• Blood bubbling from the wound

• Gasping

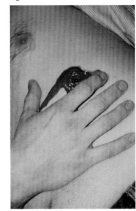

Figure 11.10 A penetrating chest injury.

 First Aid for Penetrating Chest Injuries

Check:

• Check the scene for danger.

• If it is safe to do so, check the person.

Call:

- Have someone call EMS/9-1-1. If you are alone, call EMS/9-1-1 yourself, then return to care for the person.

Care:

- Make sure ABCs are present.

Secondary Survey:

Perform a secondary survey and treat any non-life-threatening injuries:

NOTE:

Remember your gloves and other barrier devices.

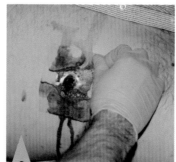

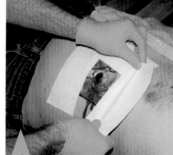

1 Have the person rest in a comfortable position.

2 Cover the wound with a dressing that will stop air from getting into the chest, such as a piece of plastic wrap or a plastic bag.

3 Tape the dressing in place but leave the side closest to the ground open to allow for drainage. This method stops air from going into the chest cavity through the wound when the person breathes in but lets it escape when the person breathes out.

4 If breathing becomes difficult after applying the dressing, you may have to raise the open side to let trapped air escape.

Continual Care:

Provide continual care until EMS personnel arrive.

Splints and Slings

Check the scene

Call for help

 Care

Secondary Survey: Perform a secondary survey and treat any non-life-threatening injuries:
Treat the injury using the RICE method

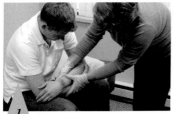

1 **R**est: Have the person stop what he was doing.

2 **I**mmobilize: Immobilize the injured area in the position that you found it.

3 **C**old: Cool the affected area for 20 minutes of every hour for the first 24 to 48 hours. If you use ice, put a thin cloth or pad between it and the bare skin.

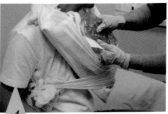

4 **E**levate: Keep the injured area above the level of the heart if possible. Do not raise the injured area if it will cause pain.

Canadian Red Cross   1-877-356-3226 | www.redcross.ca

Splints and Slings

▶ Splinting Guidelines

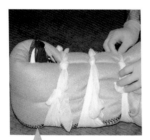

Soft splints include blankets, towels, pillows, etc.

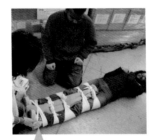

Anatomical splints use another body part for support.

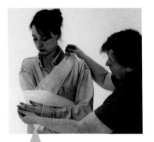

Slings are looped around the neck to support an arm, hand, or wrist.

Wound Care & Bandaging

When treating a wound:

Use non-latex **GLOVES**. If non-latex gloves are not available, use some other kind of barrier between your hands and the wound. If possible have the injured person use his/her own hands.

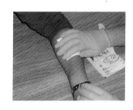

If there is much bleeding, put **DIRECT PRESSURE** on the wound until it stops.

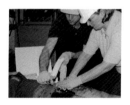

If it is a minor wound, wash the wound thoroughly with soap and water.

Wound Care & Bandaging

Check the scene
Call for help

 Care

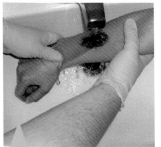

1 If possible, **RINSE** the wound for five minutes with clean, running water.

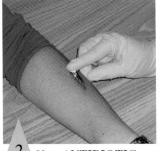

2 If an **ANTIBIOTIC** ointment or cream is available, put it on the wound as recommended by a pharmacist. (Do not apply the ointment or cream if the person has sensitivities to antibiotics.)

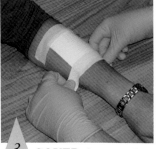

3 **COVER** the wound with a sterile dressing and/or bandage. If blood soaks through a dressing, put another one on top; don't remove the dressing next to the skin.

Canadian Red Cross   1-877-356-3226 | www.redcross.ca

PNEUMOTHORAX AND HEMOTHORAX

Chest injuries can lead to two conditions that can make breathing difficult: pneumothorax and hemothorax (Figure 11.11).

▶ Causes of Pneumothorax and Hemothorax

Pneumothorax is a condition in which air enters the chest cavity from the wound site but doesn't enter the lung. The air in the chest cavity presses against the lung, causing it to collapse.

Hemothorax is a condition in which blood accumulates in the chest cavity from the wound site but doesn't get into the lung. Because blood takes up space in the chest cavity, the lung can't expand effectively.

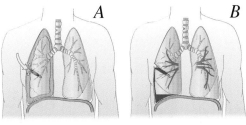

Figure 11.11 Pneumothorax (A) and hemothorax (B).

▶ Preventing Pneumothorax and Hemothorax

See "Preventing Penetrating Chest Injuries" on page 121.

▶ Signs and Symptoms of Pneumothorax and Hemothorax

See "Signs and Symptoms of Penetrating Chest Injuries" on page 121.

First Aid for Pneumothorax and Hemothorax

Treat any open wound as outlined previously.

BLUNT CHEST INJURIES

Blunt chest injuries are caused by a direct blow to the chest, but they do not result in a hole in the chest wall (Figure 11.12).

▶ Causes of Blunt Chest Injuries

- Motor vehicle collisions

- Falls

- Sports injuries

- Other crushing forces that do not create a wound in the chest wall

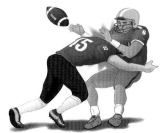

Figure 11.12 A blunt chest injury.

Preventing Blunt Chest Injuries

See "Preventing Penetrating Chest Injuries" on page 121.

 Signs and Symptoms of Blunt Chest Injuries

- Pain
- Deformity or swelling
- Bruising at the site
- Shock
- Guarded, shallow breathing

First Aid for Blunt Chest Injuries

Check:

- Check the scene for danger.
- If it is safe to do so, check the person.

Call:

- Have someone call EMS/9-1-1. If you are alone, call EMS/9-1-1 yourself, then return to care for the person.

Care:

- Make sure ABCs are present.

Secondary Survey:

Perform a secondary survey and treat any non-life-threatening injuries:

1. Keep the head and spine as still as possible as a blow to the chest may have caused head, neck, or spine injuries.

Continual Care:

Provide continual care until EMS personnel arrive.

FLAIL CHEST

Flail chest is a condition in which the chest wall becomes unstable (Figure 11.13).

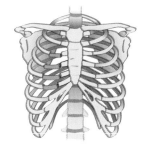

Figure 11.13 Flail chest.

▶ Causes of Flail Chest

- Fractures of the breastbone
- Fractures of the cartilage connecting the ribs to the breastbone
- Fractures of the ribs

▶ Signs and Symptoms of Flail Chest

- Difficulty breathing
- Painful breathing
- Crunching or grinding sounds in the chest
- Uneven rising of the chest during breathing
- Bruising on the chest
- Deformity or swelling
- Shock

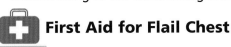 First Aid for Flail Chest

Check:

- Check the scene for danger.
- If it is safe to do so, check the person.

Call:

- Have someone call EMS/9-1-1. If you are alone, call EMS/9-1-1 yourself, then return to care for the person.

Care:

- Make sure ABCs are present.

Secondary Survey:

Perform a secondary survey and treat any non-life-threatening injuries:

1. Treat this injury as a blunt chest injury.

2. To help the person breathe better, give the person something bulky (such as a towel) to hold against the chest.

3. Keep the person still in case there are broken ribs.

Continual Care:

Provide continual care until EMS personnel arrive.

BURNS

Burns are injuries caused by chemicals, electricity, heat, or radiation.

 Preventing Burns

Chemical burns:

- Store chemicals in their original containers.
- Wear protective gear when you are handling chemicals.
- Wash your hands after touching chemicals.
- Get trained in the Workplace Hazardous Materials Information System (WHMIS).
- Follow WHMIS, MSDS, and first aid labels on packages.
- Read the label before you use a product.

Electrical burns:

- Keep electrical appliances away from water.
- If an electrical cord is frayed, fix it or get rid of it.
- If you have young children, cover electrical outlets.

Burns from lightning strikes:

- As soon as you see or hear a storm, stop swimming or boating and get away from the water because water conducts electricity.
- Go inside the closest building. If there is no building nearby, get inside a car and roll up the windows.
- Stay away from the telephone, except in an emergency. If you are caught outside, stay away from telephone poles and tall trees.
- Stay off hilltops and try to crouch down in a ravine or valley if shelters are not available nearby.
- Stay away from farm equipment and small metal vehicles such as motorcycles, bicycles, and golf carts.
- Stay away from wire fences, clotheslines, metal pipes and rails, and other things that conduct electricity.
- If you are with a group of people, stay several metres apart from each other.

Thermal burns:

- Keep matches away from children.

- Store gasoline and other highly flammable liquids outdoors.

- When you are cooking on the stove, turn the pot handles in and use only the back burners when possible.

- Keep the hot water tank temperature turned down to 49°C (120°F).

- Do not put water on a grease fire.

- Keep aerosol cans away from heat and open flames.

- Make sure your fireplace has a sturdy metal screen. Keep flammable materials away from fireplaces.

Sunburns:

- Stay out of the sun between 10:00 A.M. and 3:00 P.M., if possible.

- Wear proper clothing to protect you from too much sun.

- Use a sunscreen with a sun protection factor (SPF) of at least 15 and apply it 15 to 30 minutes before going outdoors. If you will be outdoors for a long period of time, consider using an SPF of 30. Reapply sunscreen at least every two hours and after being in the water or after vigorous activity and sweating.[1]

Fire safety:

Fires are caused by many things: heating equipment, appliances, electrical wiring, and cooking.

Make sure you have working smoke detectors in the hallway near any sleeping areas, at the top of stairs, and in every bedroom. In some provinces and territories, legislation dictates where smoke detectors must be located.

Plan and practise a fire escape route with your family.

- Sketch a floor plan of your home that shows all the rooms, doors, windows, and hallways.

[1] Adapted from www.cancer.ca

- Draw arrows that show how to escape from each room. If possible, show two ways to get out of each room. Planning to escape sleeping areas is most important because most fires happen at night.

- Plan where everyone will meet after leaving the building.

- Assign someone to call the fire department after leaving the burning building.

- When you travel, take a moment to find out the local emergency number and keep it on hand.

- If you stay in a hotel, learn escape routes and emergency procedures in case of a fire.

To escape from a fire:

- If there is smoke, crawl to get out of the building.

- Make sure children can open windows, go down a ladder, or lower themselves to the ground. Practise with them.

- Get out quickly and never return to a burning building.

- If you cannot get out, stay in the room. Stuff towels, rags, or clothing around doors and vents. If you have access to water, wet these materials first. If there is a phone, call EMS/9-1-1, even if rescuers are already outside, and tell the dispatcher exactly where you are.

 First Aid for Burns

Call EMS/9-1-1 immediately if:

- Burns make it hard for the person to breathe

- Burns cover more than one body part

- Burns result from chemicals, explosions, or electricity

Table 11.1 *First Aid by Type of Burn*

Types	Causes	First Aid
Chemical burns **NOTE:** *If the chemical is dry, brush it off the skin carefully.*	Wet or dry chemicals	**Check:** • Check the scene for danger. • If it is safe to do so, check the person. **Call:** • Call EMS/9-1-1 if the burn covers a large area of the body. **Care:** • Make sure ABCs are present. **Secondary Survey:** Perform a secondary survey and treat any non-life-threatening injuries: 1. Protect yourself by wearing protective equipment. 2. Flush the affected areas with large amounts of cool running water for at least 15 minutes. Flush the chemicals away from areas of the body that have not been contaminated. 3. Have the person remove any contaminated clothing. **Continual Care:** Seek medical attention. Refer to the appropriate Material Safety Data Sheet (MSDS) or call your local Poison Control Centre for first aid measures.

Types	Causes	First Aid
Electrical burns	Electricity Lightning	**Check:** • Check the scene for danger. • If it is safe to do so, check the person. **Call:** • Have someone call EMS/9-1-1. If you are alone, call EMS/9-1-1 yourself, then return to care for the person. **Care:** • Make sure ABCs are present. Electricity and lightning may affect the heart, so monitor the ABCs closely. **Secondary Survey:** Perform a secondary survey and treat any non-life-threatening injuries: 1. Treat the person as if she might have a spine or head injury. 2. Look for two burns (the entry and exit points). They will be open wounds that may need to be treated. **Continual Care:** Provide continual care until EMS personnel arrive.
Thermal burns	Liquid Steam Heat Flame	Cool the burn and treat according to the level of burns (see Table 11.2).
Radiation burns	Radioactive material	Refer to WHMIS (Workplace Hazardous Materials Information System).

Table 11.2 *First Aid by Level of Burn*

Levels	Signs and Symptoms	First Aid
Superficial burns	Redness Pain Possible swelling	**Check:** • Check the scene for danger. • If it is safe to do so, check the person. **Call:** • You should not need to call EMS/9-1-1 for a superficial burn, unless the person is in a great deal of pain or becomes unconscious. **Care:** • Make sure ABCs are present. **Secondary Survey:** Perform a secondary survey and treat any non-life-threatening injuries: 1. Cool the burn with running or standing water for at least 10 to 20 minutes. If the standing water becomes warm, add more cool water. **Continual Care:** Provide continual care. Once the burning has stopped, you can apply an antibiotic ointment and watch for infection. Your pharmacist or doctor can suggest products for superficial burns such as sunburns.

Levels	Signs and Symptoms	First Aid
Partial-thickness burns	Redness Pain Possible swelling Blisters	**Check:** • Check the scene for danger. • If it is safe to do so, check the person. **Call:** • Call EMS/9-1-1 if the burn covers more than 10% of the body, the person is in a great deal of pain, or the person becomes unconscious. **Care:** • Make sure ABCs are present. **Secondary Survey:** Perform a secondary survey and treat any life-threatening injuries: 1. If the burned area covers more than 10% of the person's body, call EMS/9-1-1 and treat the person for shock. Cool only a small area at a time. Cooling the person too quickly may cause the person to go into shock. If the burned area covers less than 10% of the person's body, cool the burn with running or standing water for at least 10 to 20 minutes. If this is too painful or the area cannot be put in water, cover the burn with a cool, moist sterile dressing or clean cloth to cool it. 2. Only remove clothing that is **not** stuck to the skin. 3. After cooling the skin, cover it loosely with a dry, sterile dressing, preferably non-stick gauze. **Continual Care:** Seek medical attention.

NOTE:

A person's palm is approximately 1% of his or her body. This is a quick guide to calculate the percentage of the body burned.

Levels	Signs and Symptoms	First Aid
Full-thickness burns	Redness Pain (may not be present at the worst part of burn due to nerve damage) Possible swelling Blisters Charred or waxy, white flesh Open wound 	**Check:** • Check the scene for danger. • If it is safe to do so, check the person. **Call:** • Have someone call EMS/9-1-1. If you are alone, call EMS/9-1-1 yourself, then return to care for the person. **Care:** • Make sure ABCs are present. **Secondary Survey:** Perform a secondary survey and treat any non-life-threatening injuries: 1. If the burned area covers more than 10% of the person's body, call EMS/9-1-1 and treat the person for shock. Cool only a small area at a time. Cooling the person too quickly may cause the person to go into shock. If the burned area covers less than 10% of the person's body, cool the burn with standing water. If this is too painful or the area cannot be put in water, cover the burn with a cool, moist sterile dressing or clean cloth to cool it. 2. Only remove clothing that is **not** stuck to the skin. 3. Do not try to clean a full-thickness burn. 4. Cover the burn with a dry sterile dressing. **Continual Care:** Provide continual care until EMS personnel arrive. Have the person lie down and treat him for shock.

Special Considerations

• Don't use grease or ointments on severe burns.

• Cool partial-thickness or full-thickness burns with water only, not ice.

• Blisters are a natural cooling system. Leave them in place.

• Touch a burn only with sterile or clean dressings. Do not use absorbent cotton or pull clothes over any burned area.

• If the burn involves large areas of the head, face, hands, feet, or groin, seek medical attention.

Sudden Medical Emergencies

Sudden Medical Emergencies

You are standing in line at the bank behind a 23-year-old woman who is 8 months pregnant. Suddenly, she collapses onto the floor.

FAINTING

Fainting is a brief period of unconsciousness that happens when there isn't enough blood flowing to the brain.

▶ Causes of Fainting

- Pregnancy
- Standing in one position for too long without moving
- Pain
- Traumatic information, such as news of someone's death
- Heat
- Dehydration
- Not eating enough

▶ Prevention of Fainting

- Watch for the warning signs of fainting, such as dizziness or nausea, and sit or lie down.
- Keep hydrated and nourished.
- Wear loose clothing around the neck.
- When standing up from sitting or laying down, do so slowly.

First Aid for Fainting

Check:

- Check the scene for danger.
- If it is safe to do so, check the person.

Call:

- Call EMS/9-1-1 if the person doesn't wake up in a few minutes and/or seems to have signs and symptoms of a serious condition such as injuries, abnormally coloured skin, or difficulty breathing.

Care:

- Make sure ABCs are present.

Secondary Survey:

Perform a secondary survey and treat any non-life-threatening injuries:

1. Place the person in the recovery position so that blood can start flowing to the brain again and the airway stays open.

Continual Care:

If the person is pregnant, has a history of heart disease, or has another serious illness, seek medical attention.

DIABETIC EMERGENCIES

A ***diabetic emergency*** happens when the body cannot control the level of sugar in the blood. The blood sugar level may become too high (***hyperglycemia***) or too low (***hypoglycemia***). Hyperglycemia develops slowly, so it is less likely to be a first aid emergency.

> *NOTE:*
> *Not all people with a blood sugar emergency are diabetic.*

▶ Causes of Diabetic Emergencies

- An imbalance between two or more of the following:
  - ▶ Exercise
  - ▶ Food intake
  - ▶ Insulin production

▶ Prevention of Diabetic Emergencies

- Take your medications as prescribed.
- Check your blood sugar often, especially if you are sick or not following your normal routine.
- Keep some quick-sugar foods with you at all times.

▶ Signs and Symptoms of Diabetic Emergencies

- Changes in the level of consciousness
- Changes in behaviour, such as confusion or aggression
- Rapid breathing
- Cool, sweaty skin
- Skin that is paler than normal
- Appearance of intoxication

Some diabetics wear a MedicAlert® medical identification product (see Chapter 2).

You don't need to know the difference between the two types of diabetic emergencies because first aid is the same for both.

First Aid for Diabetic Emergencies

Check:

- Check the scene for danger.
- If it is safe to do so, check the person.

Call:

- Call EMS/9-1-1 if the person is **unconscious**.

Care:

- Make sure ABCs are present.

Secondary Survey:

Perform a secondary survey and treat any non-life-threatening injuries.

If the person is **conscious** (and the person knows it is a diabetic emergency):

1. Offer the person a sugary drink such as orange or apple juice.

2. If you don't see any improvement within five minutes or the condition worsens, call EMS/9-1-1.

3. If the person's condition improves, recommend having a complete meal.

If the person is **unconscious:**

1. Perform a secondary survey and place the person in the recovery position.

Continual Care:

Provide continual care until EMS personnel arrive.

SEIZURES

A *seizure* is a temporary alteration in brain function that may produce a physical convulsion, minor physical signs, thought disturbances, or a combination of signs and symptoms.

▶ Causes of Seizures

• Head injuries

• Fever

• Certain medical conditions, such as epilepsy

• Poisons (including drugs)

• Drug or alcohol withdrawal

• Heat stroke

• Certain video games or other audiovisual stimulation that involves flashes

• Infection

▶ Preventing Seizures

• Follow the guidelines throughout this manual for preventing injuries at work, home, or play.

• If you have epilepsy, take your prescribed medication regularly.

• If your child has a fever, make sure it doesn't get too high. If a child's fever is higher than a fever caused by a normal cold or flu, see a doctor.

• Limit the amount of time spent playing video games.

Signs and Symptoms of Seizures

- A sense of urgency to get to safety

- Hallucinations such as seeing, hearing, tasting, or smelling something that doesn't actually exist

- Appearance of daydreaming

- Uncontrollable muscle movement

 ## First Aid for Seizures

Check:

- Check the scene for danger.

- If it is safe to do so, check the person.

Call:

- See below for when to call EMS/9-1-1.

Care:

During the seizure:

 1 Never put anything in the mouth.

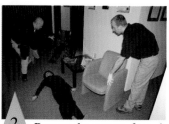
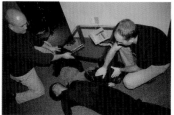

2 Protect the person from injury by:

- Moving furniture
- Protecting the person's head with blankets
- Keeping other dangers away from the person

After the seizure:

- Makes sure ABCs are present.

Secondary Survey:

Perform a secondary survey and treat any non-life-threatening injuries:

1. Make sure there aren't any fluids in the mouth.

Continual Care:

Provide continual care.

Call EMS/9-1-1 if:

- The seizure lasts more than a few minutes
- The person has several seizures in a row
- The person appears to be injured
- You are not sure what caused the seizure
- The person is pregnant
- The person is diabetic
- The person is a baby or a child
- The seizure takes place in water
- The person doesn't wake up after the seizure

 First Aid for a Baby or Child With a Fever Over 39°C (102°F)

Young children or babies with a high fever can have seizures. In most cases these are not life-threatening and they do not last long. To prevent seizures:

1. Give the child medication recommended by your doctor to reduce the fever.

2. Give the child a sponge bath with water that is room temperature (not icy cold).

3. Provide continual care.

Since these steps only temporarily lower the temperature, seek medical attention.

EMERGENCY CHILDBIRTH

 ## Causes of Emergency Childbirth

- Premature labour
- Falls
- Stress
- Trauma to the body

Signs and Symptoms of Impending Childbirth

- Contractions are two minutes apart or less
- The woman says that the baby is coming
- The baby's head is showing

Expectant Mothers

Good prenatal care starts even before your baby is conceived. Get your body in shape for pregnancy by reaching your ideal weight, getting plenty of rest, seeing a healthcare professional regularly, and making sure you have been immunized against diseases such as rubella (German measles).

When you become pregnant, follow your obstetrician's or midwife's advice about nutrition, exercise, and other good health habits.

 ## First Aid for Emergency Childbirth

Check:

- Check the scene for danger.
- If it is safe to do so, check the woman.

Call:

- Have someone call EMS/9-1-1. If you are alone, call EMS/9-1-1 yourself, then return to care for the woman.

Care:

- Make sure ABCs are present.

During labour:

1 Help the woman to be as comfortable and calm as possible.

2 Time the contractions and give this information to EMS personnel when they arrive.

3 Have the woman remove her underwear and any clothing that may be in the way of delivery.

4 Wash your hands.

5 Put clean towels, a blanket, or any available material under her buttocks.

6 Have someone stay at the woman's head and be ready to turn the woman's head and keep the airway clear if she vomits.

> **NOTE:**
> *Give the woman as much privacy as possible.*

> **NOTE:**
> *Throughout the process continue to give encouragement and reassurance.*

During birth:

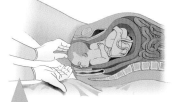

1 As the baby's head comes out, support it with one hand.

2 The baby might be in a bag of water. If the bag has not broken and is still covering the baby's head, gently tear it open with your fingers and clean it away from the baby's nose and mouth.

3 If the umbilical cord is wrapped around the baby's neck, gently loosen and unwrap it.

4 Keep the baby's mouth and nose clean of mucus and fluids by wiping them with a clean cloth.

5 Once the shoulders come out, be prepared for the rest of the baby to come out very quickly. Do not pull on the baby.

6 When the baby's feet are out, carefully hold the baby face down with the feet slightly raised. Newborns are slippery, so hold the baby firmly but do not squeeze.

7 If the baby is not breathing within 30 seconds of delivery, gently massage the baby's back. Then, if the baby is still not breathing, snap your finger against the soles of the baby's feet.

> **NOTE:**
> *Remember your gloves and other barrier devices.*

Be prepared to start CPR (see Chapter 7) or rescue breathing (for healthcare providers) (see Chapter 8) if snapping your finger against the soles of the baby's feet doesn't start it breathing.

After birth:

1 Keep the mother warm.

2 Leave the cord in place and do not pull on it. Tie the cord while you wait for the placenta to be delivered. Use two strips of sterile cloth tied tightly, one 10 cm (4 in) and one 15 cm (6 in) away from the baby.

3 Keep the baby warm by drying the baby; wrapping the baby in a clean cloth, blanket, or article of clothing; and putting the baby on the mother's abdomen or holding the baby yourself. Do not try to wash the baby.

4 The placenta, a bloody sac, will be delivered after the baby. It is normal for women to bleed until the placenta is delivered.

5 Let the placenta and cord drop onto a clean towel and keep this near the baby.

6 Gently massage the lower abdomen. This can help slow bleeding.

7 If the mother keeps bleeding, you may need to apply gentle pressure to any bleeding tears. Once the bleeding is controlled, put a sanitary pad over the mother's vaginal opening. Never place anything in the vagina.

Continual Care:

Provide continual care for both mother and baby until EMS personnel arrive.

MISCARRIAGE

Miscarriage is the spontaneous termination of a pregnancy in the first 20 weeks after conception. The risk of miscarriage drops as the pregnancy progresses.

Causes of Miscarriage

There are a number of causes of miscarriage. Some of these include:

- Hormonal or genetic reasons
- Certain illnesses
- Abnormalities in the womb
- Age
- Infection
- Trauma

Preventing Miscarriage

- Talk to your doctor about what you can do to reduce the risks of a preventable miscarriage.

Signs and Symptoms of Miscarriage

- Anxiety
- Vaginal bleeding
- Cramp-like pain that is similar to labour or menstruation

 ## First Aid for Miscarriage

Check:

- Check the scene for danger.
- If it is safe to do so, check the woman.

Call:

- Have someone call EMS/9-1-1. If you are alone, call EMS/9-1-1 yourself, then return to care for the woman.

Care:

- Make sure ABCs are present.

Secondary Survey:

Perform a secondary survey and treat any non-life-threatening injuries.

Continual Care:

Provide continual care until EMS personnel arrive.

NOTES:

Environmental Emergencies

Environmental Emergencies

A 55-year-old moose hunter has a few drinks to keep warm while he is out in the woods on an October afternoon. On his way back to his cabin, he slips and falls in a creek. It takes him more than two hours to get back. When he arrives he is shivering, his hands and feet are numb, and he has difficulty speaking.

COLD-RELATED EMERGENCIES

FROST NIP AND FROSTBITE

Frost nip is a superficial injury caused by freezing of the skin (Figure 13.1). In a case of *frostbite*, the tissue underneath the skin freezes as well (Figure 13.2). Your extremities, such as your ears, fingers, and nose, are particularly prone to frostbite. Frostbite is often associated with hypothermia.

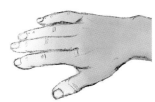

Figure 13.1 Frost nip.

 Causes of Frost Nip and Frostbite

- Exposure to cold temperatures

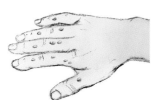

Figure 13.2 Frostbite.

 Preventing Frost Nip and Frostbite

- If you are in, on, or around a cold environment, prepare properly, wear layers of clothing, and warm yourself if you feel cold.

- Wear a hat and layers of clothing made of tightly woven fibers, such as wool, or synthetics, such as pile, which trap warm air against your body. AVOID COTTON!

- Cover up vulnerable areas such as your fingers, toes, cheeks, ears, and nose (but don't cover them too tightly).

- Drink plenty of warm fluids to help your body stay warm. If warm drinks are not available, drink plenty of plain water.

- Avoid caffeine and alcohol because they can cause dehydration, which stops your body from controlling its temperature properly.

- Take frequent breaks from the cold to let your body warm up. This will help you cope better with short periods of extreme cold.

▶ **Signs and Symptoms of Frost Nip and Frostbite**

Frost Nip:

- Pain or stinging in the area, followed by numbness

- Skin that looks paler than the area around it

Frostbite:

- Waxy skin that is colder than the area around it

- Skin that is hard and solid to the touch

- After thawing, there may be a burning sensation, redness, pain, and tenderness, and blisters may form

 First Aid for Frost Nip and Frostbite

Check:

- Check the scene for danger.

- If it is safe to do so, check the person.

Call:

- Call EMS/9-1-1 if the frost nip or frostbite is combined with severe hypothermia (see "Hypothermia", see page 151).

Care:

- Remove the person from the cold environment.

Secondary Survey:

Perform a secondary survey and treat any non-life-threatening injuries:

1. Warm the affected area gradually using warm water or body heat.

2. Don't break any blisters! Protect them with loose, dry dressings. Place gauze between the fingers or toes if they are affected.

Continual Care:

If you suspect that the person may have frostbite, seek medical attention.

Don't rub the frozen area or put snow on it. Warm the area only if you are sure it will not freeze again.

SNOW BLINDNESS

 Causes of Snow Blindness

Looking at snow for too long on a bright day can damage your eyes, causing snow blindness. That's because the snow reflects the sun's ultraviolet rays.

 Preventing Snow Blindness

- Wear sunglasses when you are outdoors in the snow in the daytime. Choose a pair that:
  - ▶ Prevents light from shining in from underneath or from above
  - ▶ Blocks more than 90% of the UV rays
  - ▶ Blocks more than 50% of the infrared rays

 Signs and Symptoms of Snow Blindness

- Redness

- Swelling of the tissue around the eyes

- Pain or a burning sensation in the eyes that may become intense

 First Aid for Snow Blindness

Check:

- Check the scene for danger.

- If it is safe to do so, check the person.

Call:

- Call EMS/9-1-1 only if you are unable to get the person to medical attention.

Care:

- Make sure ABCs are present.

Secondary Survey:

Perform a secondary survey and treat any non-life-threatening injuries:

1. Place the person in a darker environment.

2. Use cool, damp cloths to reduce pain and burning.

Continual Care:

Seek medical attention.

> The symptoms of snow blindness may not appear for several hours following exposure to bright, snowy conditions.

HYPOTHERMIA

Hypothermia is a life-threatening condition that develops when the body temperature drops too low.

 Causes of Hypothermia

• Exposure to cold temperatures for too long

People at Risk of Hypothermia:

• People who work or exercise outdoors

• Elderly people

• Young children

• People who do not consume enough calories

• People who are dehydrated

• People with health problems

• People who have had a heat-related or cold-related emergency in the past

• People who have heart disease or other conditions that cause poor circulation

• People who take medications to eliminate water from the body

 Preventing Hypothermia

• If you are in, on, or around a cold environment, prepare properly, wear layers of clothing, and warm yourself if you feel cold.

- Wear a hat and layers of clothing made of tightly woven fibers, such as wool, or synthetics, such as pile, which trap warm air against your body. AVOID COTTON!

- Cover up vulnerable areas such as your fingers, toes, cheeks, ears, and nose (but don't cover them too tightly).

- Cover up your head and trunk because you lose most of your heat from these areas.

- Drink plenty of warm fluids to help your body stay warm. If warm drinks are not available, drink plenty of plain water.

- Avoid caffeine and alcohol because they cause dehydration, which stops your body from controlling its temperature properly.

- As soon as you start shivering, get out of the cold and let your body warm up. This will help you cope better with short periods of extreme cold.

- Be extremely careful around water. Hypothermia can occur in any body of water, warm or cold.

- If your clothes get wet when you are in the cold, change into dry clothing immediately.

▶ Things to Remember About Hypothermia

- Hypothermia can be mild, moderate, or severe.

- Hypothermia can get worse very quickly if the person is wet and the environment is cold.

- Hypothermia can slowly get worse if the person is dry but the environment is cold.

- Hypothermia can occur at any time of the year.

Table 13.1 *Signs and Symptoms of Hypothermia*

Level of Severity	Signs and Symptoms
Mild	Shivering and complaining of cold
	Numbness
	Body temperature slightly below normal
Moderate	Shivering
	Numbness
	Lack of coordination and/or speech
	Confused or unusual behaviour
	Impaired judgment
Severe	Person has stopped shivering
	Person has stopped complaining of the cold
	Numbness
	Lack of coordination and/or speech
	Confused or unusual behaviour
	Impaired judgment
	Body temperature below 30°C (86°F)
	Breathing that has slowed down or stopped
	Possible unconsciousness
	Body that feels stiff

> **NOTE:**
> *Normal body temperature is 37°C (98.6°F).*

—37
—36 Mild
—35
—34 Moderate
—33
—32
—31
—30 Severe
—29
—28
—27
°C

 First Aid for Hypothermia

Check:

- Check the scene for danger.
- If it is safe to do so, check the person.

> **NOTE:**
> ***For Healthcare Providers:*** *Someone who has moderate or severe hypothermia will have a slow and irregular pulse.*

Call:

• Call EMS/9-1-1 for severe hypothermia.

Care:

1. Make sure ABCs are present.

2. Treat the person very gently and monitor breathing carefully.

3. Get the person away from the cold and into some kind of shelter, if possible.

4. Remove any wet clothing and dry the person.

5. Warm the person by wrapping him or her in blankets or putting on dry clothing. Cover the head and neck. Warm the person slowly. Warming too quickly can cause heart problems.

6. If hot water bottles, heating pads, or other heat sources are available, put them in each armpit, the groin, and the back of the neck. If you use a heating pad, make sure the person is dry. Keep a blanket, towel, or clothing between the heat source and the skin to avoid burns. Active re-warming should be used only when the person is far from a medical facility.

7. If the person is alert, give him or her warm liquids to drink (no alcohol or caffeine).

Secondary Survey:

Perform a secondary survey and treat any non-life-threatening injuries.

Continual Care:

Provide continual care until EMS personnel arrive.

FREEZING TO METAL OBJECTS

The tongue, lips, and other parts of your skin can freeze to cold metal objects.

 Causes of Freezing to Metal Objects

• Freezing of moist skin to a cold metal object

Diabetic Emergencies

 Signs and Symptoms of Diabetic Emergencies

- Changes in the level of consciousness
- Rapid breathing
- Cool, sweaty skin
- Skin that is paler than normal
- Appearance of intoxication
- Changes in behaviour, such as confusion or aggression
- A MedicAlert® product

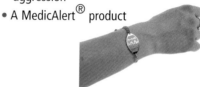

Check the scene

Call for help

 Care

If the person is **conscious** (and the person knows it is a diabetic emergency):

1. Offer the person a sugary drink such as orange or apple juice.
2. If you don't see any improvement within five minutes or the condition worsens, call EMS/9-1-1.
3. If the person's condition improves, recommend having a complete meal.

If the person is **unconscious**:

1. Perform a secondary survey and place the person in the recovery position.

Continual Care:

Provide continual care until EMS personnel arrive.

 Canadian Red Cross   1-877-356-3226 | www.redcross.ca

Seizures

In most cases seizures are not life-threatening and do not last long. Protect the person from injury by:

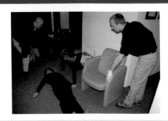

- Moving furniture
- Protecting the person's head with blankets
- Keeping other dangers away from the person

Baby or Child With a Fever Over 39°C (102°F)

Check the scene

Call for help

 Care

Young children or babies with high a fever can have seizures.

To prevent seizures in a child with a fever:

1. Give the child medication recommended by your doctor to reduce the fever.

2. Give the child a sponge bath with water that is room temperature (not icy cold).

3. Provide continual care.

Since these steps only temporarily lower the temperature, seek medical attention.

 Canadian Red Cross   1-877-356-3226 | www.redcross.ca

Poisons

Swallowed

Signs and symptoms

Burns around the mouth
Increased saliva production
Cramps and vomitting
Burning sensation in the mouth,
throat, or stomach

Check the scene
Call for help

 Care: Only induce vomitting if told to do so by the Poison Control Centre

Inhaled

Signs and symptoms

Breathing difficulties
Irritated eyes, nose, or throat
Bluish colour around the mouth

Check the scene
Call for help

 Care: Protect yourself from the poison

Get the person to fresh air

 Canadian Red Cross   1-877-356-3226 | www.redcross.ca

Poisons

▶ Injected

Signs and symptoms
> Puncture wound
> Redness and swelling around
> the entry point
> Breathing difficulties
> Prescription medications or
> drugs nearby

Check the scene
Call for help

 Care: Watch for signs of allergic reactions

▶ Absorbed

Signs and symptoms
> Hives
> Swelling
> Burning or itching
> Blisters
> Burns

Check the scene
Call for help

Care:

For all poisonings, continue to monitor the ABCs. If there is a change, call EMS/9-1-1.

▶ *1* Remove the substance from the skin.

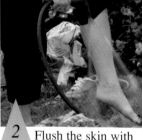

2 Flush the skin with large amounts of water for at least 15 minutes. To prevent any further injury, make sure the water flushes away from any unaffected areas of the body.

 Canadian Red Cross   1-877-356-3226 | www.redcross.ca

First Aid for Freezing to Metal Objects

Check:

- Check the scene for danger.

- If it is safe to do so, check the person.

Call:

- Call EMS/9-1-1 if you cannot safely remove the body part from the object.

Care:

1. Make sure ABCs are present.

2. Pour warm water on the surface of the object and/or the skin that is stuck to the object. Do not use hot water!

3. Gradually and gently help release the person from the metal object.

Secondary Survey:

Perform a secondary survey and treat any non-life-threatening injuries:

1. Treat the torn skin as an open wound.

Continual Care:

Provide continual care.

HEAT-RELATED EMERGENCIES

▶ Causes of Heat-Related Emergencies

Causes/risk factors can be broken into four areas[1]:

1. Illnesses:

    - Heart disease

    - Certain skin, hormone, or nervous system diseases

    - Extensive burns

    - Dehydration

2. Behaviour:

    - Spending too much time in the heat or sun

    - Not drinking enough fluids to replace the water you lose by sweating (Figure 13.3)

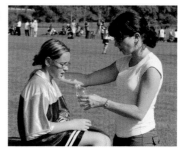

Figure 13.3 Drink plenty of cool fluids.

[1]Heat Exhaustion and Heatstroke by Amy Kunihiro, ME, available at www.emedicine.com

- Working or exercising too much in hot weather

3. Certain drugs that increase the risk of heat-related emergencies

4. Other risk factors:

   - Salt depletion or water depletion

   - Obesity

▶ **Preventing Heat-Related Emergencies**

- Drink plenty of cool fluids—this is the most important action you can take to prevent heat-related emergencies.

- Avoid being outdoors during the hottest part of the day.

- Slow down your activities as it gets hotter and don't work or exercise for too long at a time.

- Take frequent breaks in a cool or shaded area to let your body cool off. This will help you cope better with short periods of extreme heat.

- Dress for the heat and for your activity level.

- Wear a hat when you're in the sun. Wear light-coloured cotton clothing to absorb sweat and let air circulate and heat escape.

- Avoid caffeine and alcohol because they can cause dehydration, which stops your body from controlling its temperature properly.

NOTE:

People at risk of heat-related emergencies are the same as those who are at risk of cold-related emergencies.

Table 13.2 *Signs, Symptoms, and First Aid for Heat-Related Emergencies*

Type of Injury	Signs and Symptoms	First Aid	
Heat cramps	Mild muscle contractions that can become severe, usually in the legs and abdomen but can be in other body parts Normal body temperature (37°C or 98.6°F) in most cases Moist skin	**Check:** • Check the scene for danger. • If it is safe to do so, check the person. **Call:** • Call for someone to get cool water. **Care:** 1. Make sure ABCs are present. 2. Have the person rest in a cool place. 3. Give the person fluids to drink, preferably juices or sports drinks. **Secondary Survey:** Perform a secondary survey and treat any non-life-threatening injuries: 1. Gently stretch and massage the cramped muscles. **Continual Care:** Provide continual care.	47 46 45 44 43 42 41 40 39 38 37 Heat cramps °C

Type of Injury	Signs and Symptoms	First Aid
Heat exhaustion	Normal or slightly raised body temperature Moist skin Skin that is redder or paler than normal Nausea Dizziness and weakness Exhaustion	**Check:** • Check the scene for danger. • If it is safe to do so, check the person. **Call:** • Call EMS/9-1-1 if the person is vomiting or is losing consciousness. **Care:** 1. Make sure ABCs are present. 2. Have the person rest in a cool place. 3. Have the person loosen any tight clothing and if you are fanning the person remove any clothing that is soaked with sweat. 4. Put cool water on the skin and fan the person to increase evaporation. Avoid using any other substances on the skin. 5. If the person is conscious, have him take sips of cool water. **Secondary Survey:** Perform a secondary survey and treat any non-life-threatening injuries. **Continual Care:** Don't let the person do any more activities in the heat that day. If the condition gets worse, follow the treatment for heat stroke.

Heat exhaustion

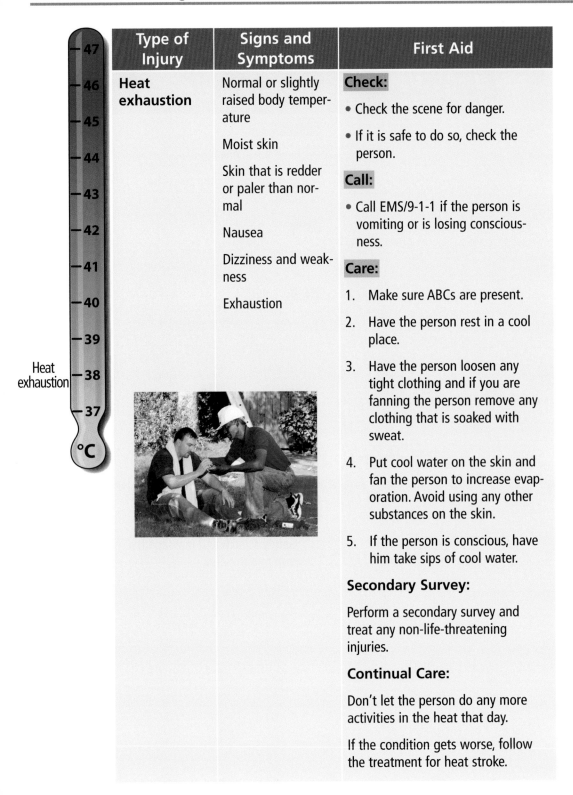

Type of Injury	Signs and Symptoms	First Aid	
Heat stroke	High body temperature, often as high as 41°C (106°F) Red, hot, dry skin, especially in the elderly Irritable, bizarre, or aggressive behaviour Progressive loss of consciousness Rapid, weak pulse becoming irregular Rapid, shallow breathing Seizures	**Check:** • Check the scene for danger. • If it is safe to do so, check the person. **Call:** • Have someone call EMS/9-1-1. If you are alone, call EMS/9-1-1 yourself, then return to care for the person. **Care:** 1. Make sure ABCs are present. 2. Have the person rest in a cool place. 3. Cool the body any way you can. Sponge the entire body with tepid or cool water, fan the person, or put covered ice packs in the groin, in each armpit, and on the back of the neck to cool large blood vessels. **Secondary Survey:** Perform a secondary survey and treat any non-life-threatening injuries. **Continual Care:** Provide continual care until EMS personnel arrive.	47 46 45 44 43 42 41 Heat stroke 40 39 38 37 °C

Heat-related emergencies will get worse without treatment and can change from one level to another very quickly.

NEAR-DROWNING

▶ Causes of Near-Drowning

• Being submerged in water, which does not allow oxygen to get into the lungs or body

▶ Preventing Near-Drowning

• Check the water depth before you swim or dive.

• Be prepared before you go in or on water. Bring any safety equipment you need.

• Know what to do to stay safe in, on, and around the water.

• Supervise children in or around all water.

• Take Canadian Red Cross water safety lessons.

▶ Signs and Symptoms of Near-Drowning

• Struggling and panicking in the water

First Aid for Near-Drowning

Check:

• Check the scene for danger.

• If it is safe to do so, check the person.

Call:

• Have someone call EMS/9-1-1. If you are alone, call EMS/9-1-1 yourself, then return to care for the person.

NOTE:

For Healthcare Providers: If you have special training, you can start rescue breathing while the person is still in the water if it does not delay removing the person from the water.

Care:

• Remove the person quickly and safely from the water but do not put yourself in danger. Try to use a reaching assist while you stay in a safe position (see Chapter 3).

Secondary Survey:

Perform a secondary survey and treat any non-life-threatening injuries.

Continual Care:

Provide continual care until EMS personnel arrive.

POISONS

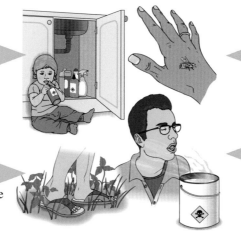

Swallowed (ingested) poisons come in contact with the mouth or lips.

Injected poisons enter the body through bites or stings or as drugs injected with a needle.

Absorbed poisons get into the body through the skin. Chemicals and plants can cause this type of poisoning.

Inhaled poisons are breathed into the body.

▶ Preventing Poisonings

- Keep all medications, household products, poisonous plants, and other toxic substances well out of the reach of children. Use locked cupboards or special child-resistant latches.

- Treat all household or drugstore products as if they could be dangerous.

- Use child-resistant safety caps on medications and other products.

- Never call medicine "candy" to persuade a child to take it.

- Keep products in their original containers with their original labels.

- Use poison symbols to identify dangerous substances and teach children what the symbols mean.

- Carefully dispose of outdated medications by giving them to the pharmacist.

- When you're using chemicals that might be dangerous, work in a well-ventilated area and follow the instructions on the package carefully.

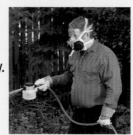

- Wear proper protective clothing any time you may come into contact with a poisonous substance.

- Keep the local Poison Control Centre number by your telephone.

Preventing Poisoning in the Workplace:

About one-quarter of all workers are exposed to chemical hazards in their workplace.

According to WHMIS regulations, employers must:

• Clearly label hazardous materials, including all toxic substances

• Tell employees about risks and precautions

• Have a detailed Material Safety Data Sheet (MSDS) available for every hazardous substance in the workplace

• Give workers who may be exposed to hazardous materials the proper training in safety measures and emergency procedures

Employees Should:

• Check all warning labels, tags, and posters in the workplace and follow the instructions carefully

• Read labels and MSDSs to find out the risks of each hazardous material, the safety measures to prevent poisoning, and the first aid for poisoning

• Never use a product that is in an unidentified bottle

Many everyday substances can be poisonous in large enough quantities.

▶ Signs and Symptoms of Swallowed Poisons

• An open container of poison nearby

• Burns around the mouth

• Increased production of saliva and/or saliva that is an abnormal colour

• Abdominal cramps and vomiting

• Seizures

• Dizziness and/or drowsiness

• Unconsciousness

• A burning sensation in the mouth, throat, or stomach

• Diarrhea

First Aid for Swallowed Poisons

Check:

- Check the scene for danger.

- If it is safe to do so, check the person.

Call:

- Call your local Poison Control Centre if the person is conscious and alert and the ABCs are fine.

- Call EMS/9-1-1 if the person has an altered level of consciousness or has difficulty breathing.

Care:

- Make sure ABCs are present.

Secondary Survey:

Perform a secondary survey and treat any non-life-threatening injuries:

1. Check the packaging of the poison, if possible, so that you know what it is.

2. Induce vomiting only if told to do so by the EMS dispatcher or the Poison Control Centre.

Continual Care:

- Provide continual care.

- If the person needs to go to hospital, bring the container as well.

▶ **Signs and Symptoms of Inhaled Poisons**

- Breathing difficulties
- Dizziness
- Seizures
- Unconsciousness
- A cloud in the air
- Irritated eyes, nose, or throat
- Vomiting
- Bluish colour around the mouth
- An unusual smell in the air

 First Aid for Inhaled Poisons

Check:

- Check the scene for danger.

• If it is safe to do so, check the person.

Call:

• Call your local Poison Control Centre if the person is conscious and alert and the ABCs are fine.

• Call EMS/9-1-1 if the person has an altered level of consciousness or has difficulty breathing.

Care:

• Get the person into fresh air, but DO NOT enter into a hazardous atmosphere yourself to do so.

Secondary Survey:

Perform a secondary survey and treat any non-life-threatening injuries.

Continual Care:

Provide continual care.

> Inhaled poisons can affect everyone in the area. Stay out of the area if you suspect that the poison may still be there.

▶ Signs and Symptoms of Injected Poisons

• Puncture wound

• Pain

• Redness and swelling at the entry point

• Problems breathing

• Prescription medications or illegal drugs nearby

First Aid for Injected Poisons

Check:

• Check the scene for danger.

• If it is safe to do so, check the person.

Call:

• Call your local Poison Control Centre if the person is conscious and alert and the ABCs are fine.

• Call EMS/9-1-1 if the person has an altered level of consciousness or has difficulty breathing.

Care:

1. Make sure ABCs are present.

2. Keep the site of the puncture lower than the heart.

3. Have the person rest in a comfortable position.

Secondary Survey:

Perform a secondary survey and treat any non-life-threatening injuries.

Continual Care:

Provide continual care.

▶ Signs and Symptoms of Absorbed Poisons

- Rash
- Burning, itching
- Swelling
- Blisters
- Hives (raised, itchy areas of skin)
- Burns
- Unconsciousness

First Aid for Absorbed Poisons

Check:

- Check the scene for danger.

- If it is safe to do so, check the person.

Call:

- Call your local Poison Control Centre if the person is conscious and alert and the ABCs are fine.

- Call EMS/9-1-1 if the person has an altered level of consciousness or has difficulty breathing.

Care:

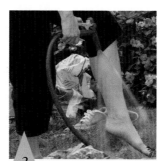

1 Make sure ABCs are present.

2 Remove the substance from the skin.

3 Flush the skin with large amounts of water for at least 15 minutes. To prevent any further injury, make sure the water flushes away from any unaffected areas of the body.

Secondary Survey:

Perform a secondary survey and treat any non-life-threatening injuries.

Continual Care:

Provide continual care.

STINGS AND INSECT BITES

 Preventing Stings and Insect Bites

When you are in wooded or grassy areas:

• Wear a long-sleeved shirt and long pants.

• Tuck your pant legs into your socks or boots and tuck your shirt into your pants. In areas with ticks, use a rubber band or tape the area where your pants meet your socks so that nothing can get underneath.

• Wear light-coloured clothing to make it easier to see tiny insects or ticks.

• Don't wear perfume.

• When you are hiking in woods and fields, stay in the middle of trails.

• Stay away from underbrush and tall grass.

• Check yourself carefully for insects or ticks after you get inside.

• If you have pets that go outdoors, spray them with repellent made for your type of pet. Check them for ticks often because your pet can bring ticks and insects into your home.

Signs and Symptoms of Stings and Insect Bites

• Pain, redness, or swelling at the site of the injury

• Insects nearby

 First Aid for Stings and Insect Bites

Check:

• Check the scene for danger.

• If it is safe to do so, check the person.

Call:

• Call EMS/9-1-1 if there are any signs of an allergic reaction.

Care:

▲*1* Make sure ABCs are present.

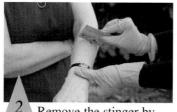

▲*2* Remove the stinger by scraping it away from the skin.

Secondary Survey:

Perform a secondary survey and treat any non-life-threatening injuries:

1. Wash the area with soap and water.

2. Apply a cold pack to help control swelling but put a thin cloth between the cold pack and the person's skin to avoid freezing the skin.

Continual Care:

Watch for signs of an allergic reaction (see Chapter 6).

If you use an insect repellent, don't use it around your lips, eyes, or any wounds or irritated skin. Follow the instructions on the label carefully. When you come inside, wash your skin with soap and water to remove the repellent. With children, do not use any insect repellents with diethyltoluamide (DEET) in concentrations greater than 25%.

First Aid for Tick Bites

Check:

• Check the scene for danger.

• If it is safe to do so, check the person.

Call:

• There is no need to call EMS/9-1-1 for a tick bite.

Care:

▲*1* Make sure ABCs are present.

▲*2* If the tick hasn't started to dig into the flesh, remove it by brushing it off the skin.

▲*3* If the tick has started to dig into the flesh, grasp its head with tweezers and pull it out. Avoid twisting the tick.

Secondary Survey:

Perform a secondary survey and treat any non-life-threatening injuries:

1. When the tick is out, wash the area with soap and water and then apply an antiseptic or antibiotic ointment to prevent infection.

2. If you cannot remove the tick or if its mouth parts stay in your skin, see a doctor.

Continual Care:

If you get a rash or flu-like symptoms within a month after the tick bite, seek medical attention (see the section on Lyme disease below).

LYME DISEASE

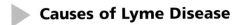 ### Causes of Lyme Disease

• A bite from an infected tick

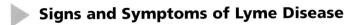 ### Signs and Symptoms of Lyme Disease

Early symptoms:

• A rash in a small red area that spreads up to 13–18 cm (5–7 in) across

• Fever, headache, weakness, and joint and muscle pain that may feel like the flu

Later symptoms (weeks or months after the bite):

• Arthritis, numbness, or a stiff neck

• Memory loss

• Problems seeing or hearing

• A high fever

• An irregular or rapid heartbeat

 ### First Aid for Lyme Disease

Seek medical attention as soon as possible.

STINGS FROM MARINE LIFE

In Canada, stings from marine life are usually from jellyfish. In other parts of the world, animals such as stingrays and sea urchins can sting you when in the water.

> **NOTE:**
>
> *None of the sea urchins in Canada are poisonous. Poisonous sea urchins can be found in other parts of the world.*

 Prevention of Stings From Marine Life

Know the water you are swimming in and stay away from stinging marine life.

 Signs and Symptoms of Stings From Marine Life

- Pain
- Redness
- Rash
- Swelling

 First Aid for Stings From Marine Life

Check:

- Check the scene for danger.
- If it is safe to do so, check the person.

Call:

- Call your local pharmacist to find the most appropriate treatment.
- Call EMS/9-1-1 if the person is having airway or breathing problems.

Care:

1. Make sure ABCs are present.

2. Bathe the area with lots of seawater or cool, salty water. Do not rub the area.

3. While wearing gloves, remove any tentacles or pieces of the animal.

4. Scrape or shave the area with a razor or the edge of a knife.

> **NOTE:**
>
> *Remember your gloves and other barrier devices.*

Secondary Survey:

Perform a secondary survey and treat any non-life-threatening injuries:

1. Put a cold pack on the area for the first hour to reduce the pain.

Continual Care:

After the area dries, apply a cream as recommended by a pharmacist.

SNAKEBITES

 Prevention of Snakebites

- Do not aggravate a snake.
- If out hiking, watch where you are stepping.
- Wear proper footwear when hiking.

 First Aid for Snakebites

Check:

- Check the scene for danger.
- If it is safe to do so, check the person.

Call:

- Call EMS/9-1-1 if you think the snake is poisonous.

Care:

1. Make sure ABCs are present.
2. Keep the injured site still and lower than the heart if possible.

Secondary Survey:

Perform a secondary survey and treat any non-life-threatening injuries:

1. Check the temperature and colour of the limb beyond the site of the bite and note if it is abnormally cold or warm compared to the other limb. Report this when you seek medical attention.

Continual Care:

If you have a physical description of the snake, report it to medical personnel because it may help them provide the best treatment.

Never treat snakebites by:

- Applying ice
- Applying suction
- Cutting the wound
- Applying a tourniquet

ANIMAL BITES

 First Aid for Animal Bites

Check:

• Check the scene for danger.

• If it is safe to do so, check the person.

Call:

• Call your local animal control department.

Care:

1. Try to get the person safely away from the animal without injuring yourself.

2. Do not try to capture the animal.

3. Control any deadly bleeding.

Secondary Survey:

Perform a secondary survey and treat any non-life-threatening injuries.

If the wound is **minor**:

1. Wash it with soap and water.

2. Control any bleeding and put a dressing on the wound.

Continual Care:

Watch later for signs and symptoms of infection (see Chapter 11).

> **NOTE:**
> *If the animal is not familiar to you or there is severe bleeding, seek medical attention.*

SUBSTANCE MISUSE AND ABUSE

Many substances, such as alcohol and drugs, can be used improperly (Figure 13.4). When these substances are misused or abused, they poison the body.

▶ **Stimulants**

• Stimulants affect your brain and nerves to speed up physical and mental activity.

• Many stimulants are taken as pills, but some can be absorbed or inhaled.

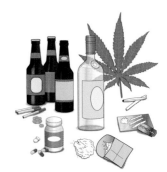

Figure 13.4 Alcohol and drugs.

▶ Hallucinogens

- Hallucinogens cause changes in mood, sensation, thought, emotion, and self-awareness.

- They can cause intense fear, panic, paranoid delusions, vivid hallucinations, deep depression, tension, and anxiety.

▶ Depressants

- Depressants send signals to your brain and nerves that slow down physical and mental activity.

- They make you drowsy and impair your coordination and judgment.

- Alcohol is the most widely used and abused depressant in Canada.

▶ Designer Drugs

- Designer drugs do not fit into any of the categories mentioned above.

- They are chemically altered versions of medical drugs, such as narcotics and amphetamines.

- The effects can be unpredictable and dangerous.

- One of the more commonly used designer drugs is "Ecstasy."

▶ Signs and Symptoms of Substance Misuse or Abuse

Like other poisons, the general signs and symptoms of substance misuse and abuse are similar to those of other medical emergencies:

- Moist or flushed skin
- Chills or fever
- Changes in breathing
- Changes in the level of consciousness

- Sweating
- Nausea or vomiting
- Seizures
- Altered mental status

✚ First Aid for Substance Misuse or Abuse

Check:

- Check the scene for danger.
- If it is safe to do so, check the person.

Call:

- Call EMS/9-1-1 if the person is having seizures, has difficulty breathing, is unconscious, or is behaving aggressively.

Care:

> **NOTE:**
> *Remember your gloves and other barrier devices.*

- Make sure ABCs are present.

Secondary Survey:

Perform a secondary survey and treat any non-life-threatening injuries:

1. You don't need to know exactly what substance the person has taken. Just look for any abnormal:

   - breathing;

   - skin colour, temperature, and moisture; or

   - behaviour.

Continual Care:

Provide continual care.

> **NOTE:**
> **For Healthcare Providers:**
> *Healthcare providers can also check for an abnormal pulse.*

ALCOHOL POISONING

Alcohol impairs your judgment, slows down your reflexes, and makes driving unsafe. Just two drinks in less than an hour can create unsafe levels of alcohol in the blood of an average 160-pound person.

Alcohol poisoning is a condition in which a toxic amount of alcohol has entered the body.

▶ Causes of Alcohol Poisoning

- Drinking excessive amounts of alcohol in a short period of time

▶ Preventing Alcohol Poisoning or Injury Due to Intoxication

- Have non-alcoholic beverages available at a party.

- Never drink and drive—this applies to boats and recreational vehicles as well as cars.

- Limit yourself to one drink per hour.

- Don't drink before a party.

- If you are angry or depressed, refrain from drinking alcohol.
- Eat plenty of food before you drink and while you are drinking.
- Avoid salty foods that may make you thirsty and encourage you to drink more.
- Do not play drinking games.

▶ Signs and Symptoms of Alcohol Poisoning

- Confusion
- Seizures
- Low body temperature
- Blue-tinged skin or skin that is paler than normal

- Vomiting
- Slow or irregular breathing
- Unconsciousness

First Aid for Alcohol Poisoning

Check:

- Check the scene for danger.
- If it is safe to do so, check the person.

Call:

- Have someone call EMS/9-1-1. If you are alone, call EMS/9-1-1 yourself, then return to care for the person.

Care:

- Make sure ABCs are present.

Secondary Survey:

Perform a secondary survey and treat any non-life-threatening injuries.

Continual Care:

Roll the person into the recovery position.

Kit Contents

Kit Contents

FIRST AID KIT

Keep a first aid kit readily available in your home, cottage, car, boat, workplace, and recreation area (Figure A.1). Store it in a dry place and replace used or outdated contents regularly.

A first aid kit should contain the following:

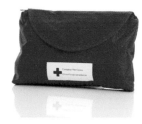

Figure A.1 A first aid kit.

❏ Emergency telephone numbers for EMS/9-1-1, your local Poison Control Centre, and your personal doctors

❏ Home and office phone numbers for family members, friends, or neighbours who can help

❏ Sterile gauze pads (dressings) in small and large squares to place over wounds

❏ Adhesive tape

❏ Roller and triangular bandages to hold dressings in place or to make an arm sling

❏ Adhesive bandages in assorted sizes

❏ Scissors

❏ Tweezers

❏ Safety pins

❏ Instant ice packs

❏ Disposable non-latex gloves, such as surgical or examination gloves

❏ Flashlight, with extra batteries in a separate bag

❏ Antiseptic wipes or soap

❏ Pencil and pad

❏ Emergency blanket

❏ Eye patches

❏ Thermometer

❏ Barrier devices, such as a pocket mask or face shield

❏ Coins for pay phone

❏ *First Aid & CPR Manual*

For more information on the different models of Canadian Red Cross First Aid kits that are available, please contact your local Red Cross office or look on our Website at www.redcross.ca.

NOTE:

Legislation dictates what type of first aid kit is required for the workplace. Go to www.redcross.ca/firstaidlegislation for more details.

EMERGENCY SUPPLIES KIT

Have supplies ready for an emergency. Store them in a backpack or a duffle bag so you can take them with you if you have to evacuate the area.

❏ Four litres of water per person per day (use sealed, unbreakable containers and replace the supply every six months). Have enough for at least three days.

❏ Packaged or canned food that won't go bad and a can opener. Replace the food once a year.

❏ Walking shoes, rain gear, and a change of clothing

❏ Blankets or sleeping bags

❏ A first aid kit and prescription medications (check the medications every six months to make sure they haven't passed their expiry date)

❏ Toilet paper and other personal supplies

❏ An extra pair of glasses

❏ A battery-powered radio and flashlight, along with extra batteries

❏ Spare cash

❏ An extra set of car keys

❏ A list of your family doctors

❏ Important family information such as a list of any medical conditions or medical devices, such as pacemakers

❏ Photocopies of all important identification for you and your family, including health card numbers

❏ Special items for babies, elderly, or disabled household members

❏ Cell phone and contact information for family and friends

EMERGENCY CAR KIT

Keep an emergency kit in your car.

❏ A battery-powered radio and flashlight, with extra batteries

❏ A blanket

❏ Booster (jumper) cables

❏ A fire extinguisher

❏ A Canadian Red Cross first aid kit

❏ Bottled water and high-energy foods that won't go bad (replace the water every six months and the food once a year)

❏ Maps of the area

❏ A shovel

❏ Flares

❏ A tire repair kit and pump

❏ Matches and a "survival" candle in a deep can that will burn for many hours

Glossary

Abdomen: The part of the body below the chest and above the pelvis. It contains the stomach, intestines, liver, spleen, and other organs.

Abdominal thrusts: A method to remove a foreign object from the airway.

Absorbed poison: A poison that enters the body through the skin.

ABCs: Airway, breathing, and circulation.

Airway: The pathway for air from the mouth and nose to the lungs.

Airway obstruction: Something in the airway that stops air from reaching the lungs.

Allergic reaction: The body's response to a substance to which it is particularly sensitive. The response can be mild or very severe.

Amputation: The complete or partial severing of a body part.

Anaphylaxis: A severe allergic reaction.

Anemia: A condition caused by a lack of red blood cells.

Angina: A cardiovascular condition in which the heart muscles need more oxygen than they are getting, causing chest pain or pressure that comes and goes. It is usually more frequent with exertion or stress.

Arteries: Large blood vessels that carry blood from the heart to the lungs and carry oxygen-rich blood from the heart to the rest of the body.

Aspiration: Inhaling blood, vomit, saliva, or foreign material into the lungs.

Avulsion: A piece of skin and sometimes other soft tissue that is torn away.

Bandage: Material used to wrap or cover a part of the body or to hold a dressing or splint in place.

Bone: The dense, hard tissue that forms the skeleton.

Brain: The centre of the nervous system that controls body functions.

Breathing emergency: A situation in which breathing is so impaired that the person's life is in danger.

Burn: An injury caused by heat, chemicals, electricity, or radiation.

Bystander: Someone who is present at the scene of a situation or emergency.

Cardiac arrest: A condition in which the heart has stopped beating or beats too irregularly or too weakly to pump blood effectively.

Cardiopulmonary resuscitation (CPR): A first aid technique that combines rescue breaths and chest compressions for someone whose breathing and heart have stopped.

Cardiovascular disease: Any disease of the heart and blood vessels. Also called heart disease.

Care: A check and immediate treatment for conditions that are an immediate threat to someone's life.

Cells: The basic units of all living tissue.

Check, Call, Care: The basic steps to follow in any emergency.

Child: Anyone between the ages of one and eight. (One to the onset of puberty for healthcare providers.)

Choking: The condition in which someone's airway is partly or completely blocked by a foreign object.

Cholesterol: A fatty substance that can cause buildup on artery walls, making the arteries narrower and restricting blood flow.

Cold-related emergency: A general term for conditions caused by being exposed to cold temperatures for too long. Includes frost nip, frostbite, and hypothermia.

Compression: Rhythmic pressure that is put on the chest to dislodge something blocking the airway or to circulate blood when the heart isn't beating effectively.

Concussion: A temporary impairment of brain function, usually caused by a blow to the head.

Consciousness: A state of awareness and responsiveness.

Consent: The permission given by the ill or injured person to the First Aider to provide care.

Continual care: Providing reassurance and follow-up care after an injury or illness.

Contraction: A squeezing action made by the muscles in the womb during labour, in preparation for childbirth.

Defibrillation: An electric shock that is given to correct a life-threatening heart rhythm.

Diabetic: A person with diabetes cannot regulate the balance between insulin and sugar.

Diabetic emergency: A condition in which a person with diabetes becomes ill because of a blood sugar level that is too high or too low.

Direct pressure: Pressure that is put on a wound to control bleeding.

Disease: An impairment of health or a condition of abnormal functioning.

Dislocation: An injury in which a bone is moved out of its normal position at a joint.

Dispatcher: The emergency medical services person who answers the emergency telephone number and decides which EMS professionals to send to the scene and who may give advice about first aid until EMS personnel arrive.

Dressing: A pad placed directly over a wound to absorb blood and other body fluids and to prevent infection.

Elevation: A technique to help slow the flow of blood to an injured area, such as a fracture, by raising the injured body part above the level of the heart.

Emergency: A situation requiring immediate action.

Emergency medical services (EMS) personnel: Trained and equipped people, including police, firefighters, and ambulance personnel, who are dispatched through a local emergency number to give emergency care to ill or injured people.

Emergency medical services (EMS) system: A network of community resources and personnel organized to give emergency care in cases of injury or sudden illness.

Epilepsy: A condition that causes seizures. It can usually be controlled by medication.

Erectile dysfunction drugs: Prescription medications such as Viagra®, Levitra®, and Cialis®, used to treat problems getting or maintaining an erection.

Exhale: To breathe air out of the lungs.

External bleeding: Bleeding from an open wound in the skin.

Fainting: A loss of consciousness caused by a temporary drop in blood flow to the brain.

Finger sweep: A technique used to remove foreign material from someone's mouth.

First aid: Immediate care given to someone who is ill or injured until more advanced care can be obtained.

First Aider: A person with some training who gives immediate care to someone who is ill or injured until more advanced care can be obtained.

Fracture: A break in bone tissue.

Frostbite: The freezing of the skin and underlying tissues of a particular body part. It is a serious condition that most often affects the fingers, toes, ears, and nose.

Frost nip: The freezing of the skin of a particular body part. It is a superficial injury that most often affects the fingers, toes, ears, and nose.

Full-thickness burn: A burn that affects both layers of skin and the tissues underneath. The skin may be charred. Also known as a third-degree burn.

Head-tilt/chin-lift: A technique for opening the airway in an unconscious adult, child, or baby.

Head-to-toe check: A thorough check for injuries or conditions that need attention and could become life-threatening or limb-threatening if they are not cared for.

Heart: The muscular organ that pumps blood through the body.

Heart attack: A sudden illness in which an artery that feeds the heart becomes blocked, stopping part of the heart muscle from getting the oxygen-rich blood that it needs.

Heat cramps: Muscle pains, usually involving the calf and abdominal muscles, caused by working or exercising in a hot environment.

Heat exhaustion: A condition that occurs when the body temperature gets too high, usually from hard work or exercise in a hot, humid environment.

Heat-related emergency: A range of conditions caused when the body temperature gets too high, usually from hard work or exercise in a hot, humid environment. It includes heat cramps, heat exhaustion, and heat stroke.

Heat stroke: A life-threatening condition that develops when the body's temperature is extremely high and the body cannot cool itself.

Hemothorax: A condition in which blood accumulates in the chest cavity from the wound site but doesn't get into the lung. Because blood takes up space in the chest cavity, the lung can't expand effectively.

Hyperglycemia: A diabetic condition in which there is too much sugar in the bloodstream.

Hypoglycemia: A diabetic condition in which there is too little sugar in the bloodstream.

Hypothermia: A life-threatening condition that develops when the body's temperature drops too low, usually from being exposed to cold temperatures for too long.

Immobilize: To use a splint or other method to keep an injured body part from moving.

Infection: A condition caused by germs such as viruses and bacteria.

Inhale: To breathe air into the lungs.

Inhaled poison: A poison that is breathed into the lungs.

Injected poison: A poison that enters the body through a bite, sting, or hypodermic needle.

Injury: Damage to the body from an external force such as a blow, fall, fire, or collision.

Insulin: A hormone the body needs to use sugar for energy.

Internal bleeding: Bleeding inside the body.

Jaw thrust: An alternative to the head-tilt/chin-lift method for opening the airway.

Joint: Where two or more bones meet.

Labour: The contractions of the womb that come before childbirth.

Laceration: A cut. The edge can be jagged or smooth.

Ligament: A fibrous band that holds bones together at a joint.

Lungs: The pair of organs that take oxygen in and remove carbon dioxide during breathing.

Lyme disease: An illness spread by infected ticks.

MedicAlert® medical identification product: A wallet card or a bracelet, watch strap, anklet, or necklace with a tag indicating that the person wearing it has a particular medical condition.

Medical emergency: An illness or condition requiring immediate medical attention.

Muscle: A soft tissue that lengthens and shortens to move body parts.

Narcotics: A group of drugs that reduce pain and induce sleep.

Nerve: A part of the nervous system that carries impulses between the brain and all body parts.

Normal breathing: A state when airways to the lungs are fully open, allowing air to easily move in and out, leading to normal breathing.

Partial-thickness burn: A burn through both layers of skin. The skin may blister and look red and wet. Sometimes called a second-degree burn.

Pelvis: The part of the body between the abdomen and the legs. It contains the intestines, bladder, and reproductive organs.

Pneumothorax: A condition in which air enters the chest cavity from the wound site, but doesn't enter the lung. The air in the chest cavity presses against the lung, causing it to collapse.

Poison: Any substance that causes injury, illness, or death when it enters the body.

Poison Control Centre: A centre staffed by medical professionals to give information about first aid in cases of poisoning. Poison Control Centre phone numbers are on the inside front page of the telephone directory.

Primary survey: An examination of the emergency scene and the ill or injured person for life-threatening conditions.

Pulse: The beat felt in arteries near the skin with each contraction of the heart.

Rescue breathing: The technique of breathing air into someone who isn't breathing.

Respiratory arrest: A condition in which breathing has stopped or isn't effective.

Respiratory distress: A condition in which breathing is difficult.

Risk factors: Conditions or behaviours that increase the chance that a person will develop a particular disease or get a particular injury.

Secondary survey: A verbal, visual, and physical check of an ill or injured person for conditions that need attention and could become life-threatening if they are not cared for.

Seizure: A temporary alteration in brain function that may produce a physical convulsion, minor physical signs, thought disturbances, or a combination of signs and symptoms.

Shaken Baby Syndrome: The type of injuries or combination of injuries a baby or child receives from being shaken.

Shock: A serious condition caused when the circulatory system cannot get enough oxygen-rich blood to all parts of the body. It can be the result of severe blood loss or an allergic reaction, among other causes.

Sign: A signal of injury or illness that a First Aider can see, feel, smell, or hear.

Skin: The membrane that covers the entire surface of the body.

Soft tissue: The layers of skin, fat, muscles, and other soft body structures.

Spinal cord: The bundle of nerves that run through the vertebrae between the brain and the lower back.

Splint: A device used to stop body parts from moving.

Sprain: The stretching and tearing of ligaments and other soft tissues at a joint.

Strain: The stretching and tearing of muscles and tendons.

Stroke: A disruption of blood flow in the brain, causing weakness and/or speech problems.

Sudden medical emergency: A sudden illness or condition that needs immediate medical attention.

Superficial burn: A burn that affects just the top layer of skin. The skin will look red and dry. Sometimes called a first-degree burn.

Swallowed (ingested) poison: A poison that enters the body by being swallowed.

Symptom: A signal of injury or illness that the ill or injured person tells you that he or she feels.

Tendon: A fibrous band that attaches muscle to bone.

Tissue: A group of cells that work together to perform specific functions.

Triage: The process of sorting and providing care to several ill or injured people according to the severity of their injuries or illnesses.

Veins: Blood vessels that carry oxygen-rich blood from the lungs back to the heart and carry oxygen-poor blood from all parts of the body back to the heart.

Ventricular fibrillation: A life-threatening condition in which the heart muscle quivers instead of pumping blood.

Ventricular tachycardia: A life-threatening condition in which the heart muscle contracts too quickly to pump enough blood to the body.

Vertebrae: The 33 bones that make up the spine.

Vital signs: Three key characteristics of someone's condition: level of consciousness, breathing, and the appearance of the skin.

Wound: An injury to soft tissues.

Index

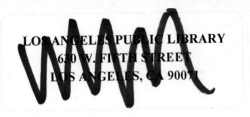
THE BOOK SUPREMACY

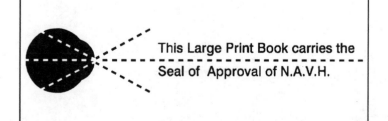